CU00859110

Institute of Clinical Acupuncture and Oriental Medicine

1270 Queen Emma Street, Suite 107
Honolulu, Hawaii 96813
Phone/Fax (808)521-2288

December 15, 2001

It is my belief that Acupuncture and Oriental Medicine offer the best hope for the future of health care. The time-tested techniques of this holistic system of medicine, whose roots are traced back over three thousand years, have given countless millions of people relief from their suffering and helped them return to a state of balanced health.

In this book, Dr. Huang has provided a look into how Oriental Medicine can help those people who suffer with arthritis, a disorder that is extremely prevalent in our society. I hope that many people will find this information valuable as they seek effective treatments for their ailments.

It is said that a great physician is one who educates the public in order to prevent the continued suffering of all people. I give my whole-hearted support to Dr. Huang for his efforts to bring this information to the world.

Sincerely,

John Welden, Dipl.Ac., L.Ac.
Dean of Academic Affairs, ICAOM

VALC

Stop Suffering from Arthritis

TCM Can Help You

Dr. Tom J. Huang, DAc. Dipl.Ac. Ch.

(NCCAOM)

Library of Congress Number: 2002090483
ISBN: Hardcover   1-4010-4770-X
                 Softcover   1-4010-4769-6

Copy Editor: Susan Valcourt

ASK YOUR DOCTOR

The material in this book is for informational purposes only. It is not
intended to serve as a prescription for you, or to replace the advice of
your medical doctor. Please discuss all aspects of your condition with
your physician before beginning any alternative program.

This book was printed in the United States of America.

To order additional copies of this book, contact:
Xlibris Corporation
1-888-795-4274
www.Xlibris.com
Orders@Xlibris.com

Tom J. Huang

Doctor of Acupuncture

Diplomate Acupuncturist

Diplomate Chinese Herbalist

Diplomate Herbologist

Dr. Tom Huang is a Doctor of Acupuncture and Herbologist and currently operates his own clinic in Honolulu, Hawaii. He is also a Diplomate, NCCAOM, and Hawaii and Florida state licensed acupuncturist.

Tom Huang

420 Nahua Ave.

Honolulu, HI 96815

(808) 922-7188 email: _tjhuang@aol.com_

Professional Experience

Institute of Clinical Acupuncture & Oriental Medicine In-structor, 1998-present.
Oriental Medical Institute of Hawaii Instructor, 1996-1998
NCCAOM Diplomate Acupuncturist and Chinese Herbalist
Hawaii state Doctor of Acupuncture and Chinese Herbologist
Florida state licensed Acupuncturist and Chinese Herbalist
Advanced Studies, Oriental Medical Institute of Hawaii
Operate and own acupuncture clinic and herb shop.

Education

University of Health Science, 2000

Oriental Medical Institute of Hawaii

Graduated, 1995

A.A. Degree

Advanced Studies

Heald Electronic College, 1983

Electronic Engineering

With Gratitude and Grateful Acknowledgment

This book is dedicated to my father, whose
wisdom and practical application led me to
pursue the avenues of healing

A Father's Wish For His Children

1. Don't jump to conclusions. Take the time to think logically before forming a judgment, acting or reacting.

2. Don't focus too much on selfish interests. Take the time to pay attention to others and what is happening around you.

3. Be reasonable and moderate in all situations. Take the example of the bamboo. It is strong, but flexible; it moves with the wind and the rain. Iron, on the other hand, is very strong, but is also brittle, and under pressure, will break.

4. Use the well-worn paths to help lead you to further discoveries. You can learn from the experiences of others, but also make your own knowledge.

5. Possess the wisdom and judgment of Solomon: have understanding of what is true and right.

6. Build your future. Expect a good outcome, and work towards it in each moment today. Your good expectations will enable its unfoldment.

7. When great demands are made upon you, stand firm, face them and do not shift away. You will discover that you have the skill, energy and vigor to focus on the situation and bring forth good fruit. If you apply enthusiastic devotion to a cause and are diligent in its furtherance, you will prevail.

Introduction

In my practice, I see many people who suffer from arthritis. Often they come to see me after traditional western medical treatment has failed to relieve their symptoms and their pain. I want to explain my experience to these people, and also to reach other people like them, to let them know that there are other choices they can make and other answers to their questions.

I don't claim to have all the solutions, but I do know that there are less invasive alternatives to today's established medical approach. It is unnecessary to further debilitate the weakened body through the use of surgery or drugs, which are conventionally prescribed by physicians. In some cases a combination of both eastern and western medicine can work together to relieve the problem.

Many books are being written today about supposed cures for arthritis. Most of these do not address the fact that there are different types of arthritis. The average person does not realize that these supposed cures are dedicated to only one brand of arthritis—a type they may or may not have! Taking the wrong "prescription" can be as bad as not seeking treatment at all.

I believe that all people have arthritis to some degree. In my opinion, osteoporosis is a form of arthritis, and is a natural process of aging. This type, indeed all of the five types of arthritis, can not only be treated, with very good results, but they can also be prevented, or at least the progression of the disease can be slowed.

If I can help to show the average person how to avoid, slow down, or even reverse the effects of arthritis, I will have fulfilled my purpose in writing this book.

You will notice that when I list the herbs used to treat the differing types of arthritis, I use the Chinese medical name for them. The reason is that if you go to a Chinese herbal shop, or seek treatment from a Chinese physician, they will recognize these scientific names immediately, and know what you are talking about. If you use the English names, the herb shop proprietor or the eastern doctor may not understand what herbs you want. In this way we can avoid misunderstandings.

Please remember that the material here is for informational purposes only. It is not intended to serve as a prescription for you, or to replace the advice of your medical doctor. Please discuss all aspects of your condition with your physician before beginning any alternative program.

Chapter 1

Know Your Opponent

What's going on? Your knees hurt. Your elbows and shoulders are stiff. Your fingers have trouble grasping small items. It seems like you just don't have any energy any more. It's hard to walk, and forget about going up and down stairs. Why is this happening?

You have arthritis.

In order to understand what is happening in your body, first we must find out more about arthritis. Just as each person is different, each type of arthritis is different. Hopefully the knowledge that you gain from reading this book can help you to understand your problems. Though this material will increase what you know about arthritis, if at any time you're wondering if you have it, please consult a medical doctor as soon as possible.

Let me introduce myself. I am a Doctor of Acupuncture and Herbologist with a practice in Honolulu, Hawaii. I have seen many different cases and different kinds of arthritis. In the treatment of my patients, I realized that many of them did not even know that they had arthritis. Some also didn't realize that they had taken bad advice, sometimes from medical professionals. I hope that you can use the information here:

1. To try to prevent arthritis;
2. To help slow the onslaught of arthritis if you have it;
3. To ease the pain instead of just suffering.

I will explain a little about Traditional Chinese Medicine (TCM), and how eastern practitioners are able to treat the individual who has the disease. You will see that the methods are quite different than what the traditional western medical professional typically prescribes, and often yield astonishing results.

You will notice that I use many Chinese medical terms that may be unfamiliar to you. If you need more explanation than what is written, please refer to the glossary at the end of the book.

To begin, let me tell you an interesting story from the Chinese Zodiac that applies to our subject. Long, long ago, when humans were the greatest hunters of the world, the animals held a meeting in the forest. All of the animals except humans were there. The animals despised the humans because humans hunted the animals and killed them, not only for food, but also for sport. So all of the animals gathered and prayed to their mighty god.

"Oh, mighty God!" the boar prayed. "Please curse the humans with digestion problems."

The boar's god heard his plea, and so the humans were given digestion problems.

"Oh mighty God!" the goat prayed, "Curse the humans so that they cannot grow fur and will be cold during the winter."

The goat's god listened to his cries, and we humans do not have thick and shaggy fur like a bear or goat, and so we are prone to catching colds.

"Oh mighty God!" the ox prayed. "Let these humans, who wish to control everything, have only two feet that are easily hurt." The ox's god heard the pious ox, and so, we humans only have two legs, and if we are not careful, we easily sprain them.

"Oh mighty God!" the mustang prayed. "Let not these smart-alec, back-stabbing human beings grow as large as I, and further, give them pain in their joints! Not only that, when the weather changes, let them feel pain such that they wish to die. And also in the mornings, let them feel stiffness and pain, especially in their joints and spine!"

The mustang's god listened to the wild mustang and granted him that plea. And as a result, we humans were cursed with these ailments.

* * *

This is, of course, just an amusing story. However, story or no, human beings have these problems. And these difficulties are very severe—they can damage our health and even our lives. We cannot run or hide from them, and all people have to face them. We might as well face them sincerely and solve the issues if we can. If we cannot solve them, we should learn a little bit more about them, or at least try and understand the real problems, their features, and their strange behavior.

There is an old Chinese saying:

If I can get it, it is my destiny.
If I cannot get it, it is my luck.

I use this attitude to face the mounting problem of arthritis.

13

VALC

Philosophy

Traditional Chinese Medicine embraces the concept that you cannot treat the whole individual by treating his individual parts. In order to understand and care for a person and his problems, we must evaluate his entire system. The body consists of many complicated inter-reacting components, and we must take these into consideration when trying to find the reasons for its difficulties.

If a tree's leaves are disfigured, we may cut off those leaves to try to cure the problem. When the new leaves grow the same way, we find out this was not the solution. The underlying reason for the misshapen leaves could be the result of one factor, or of multiple factors, including root damage, pests, lack of water, etc.

Life and Air

Sunshine, water and air are vital for human life. Air is especially important. A person will lose consciousness within five minutes if deprived of oxygen. After nine minutes without oxygen, brain cells begin to die. From this we understand how important air is.

Unfortunately, we live in a world inundated with air pollution, and because of this we absorb many sorts of contaminants or microorganisms that can damage our organs. In human beings these poisons can cause obstructed airway, bronchitis, bronchial asthma, pulmonary disease, emphysema, and other not-so-obvious effects. In this context, obstructed airway refers to the swelling of membranes in the throat that occurs when it is irritated for whatever reason.

What is the solution? Reduce inflammation, improve environment, emphasize education, normalize airway, and practice T'ai Chi, or Chi Kung. Strengthen your yuan qi (pronounced chee), your body's foundation.

Hold it! What am I talking about? Here's your first introduction to Chinese medicine. Yuan qi, your body's foundation, is made up of your inherited constitution plus fuel and air. Practitioners of Traditional Chinese Medicine (TCM) believe your kidneys hold the blueprint of your inherited physical nature. This is called kidney essence, or *qi*. To build your foundation, you add *gu qi* (fuel) and atmosphere *qi* (air) to your kidney essence. All together these elements make up your *yuan qi*.

According to TCM, your kidneys hold the source, or power, of your being. Therefore, to remain healthy, you must increase your power (your *yuan qi*) through enhancing your external input (food and air) and strengthening your kidney function.

Without a strong kidney function (foundation), your body cannot carry out its vital functions of warming, sealing, evaporating, promoting, and protecting. What does this mean?

Warming means keeping your body temperature constant and correct.

Sealing refers to sealing in your vital fluids and essence—your blood, your moisture, your power—just like in an engine, keeping your gaskets tight.

Evaporation refers to the dispersion of the fluids you have taken in, i.e. through perspiration or urination.

Promoting deals with your circulation functions.

Protecting, of course, refers to your immune system functions.

The Western medical approach is often to treat the symptoms of disease rather than identifying and eliminating the underlying problems. In the process, sometimes the body becomes more debilitated, through the use of surgery or medication. These "cures" may take care of the symptoms, but often create others (side effects), and new drugs or more surgery might be prescribed to take care of the new symptoms.

Here is an example of what I am talking about. A building holds a group of terrorists who have heavy artillery. Western law enforcement arrives and begins bombing the building. The terrorists are killed, but the building is destroyed. Taking the opposite approach, in this example, eastern law enforcement would begin to negotiate. If negotiations failed, non-lethal weapons would be used. The problem is solved and the building is still in one piece. This explains the concept of eastern treatment compared to western medication.

Another important concept of eastern treatment is that since each body is different and since diseases are constantly mutating to fool our immune systems, we must re-diagnose and give a new herb "prescription" after each treatment of the patient. We don't use the same treatment in every case.

Circulation of Blood and Energy

A person's inner *qi* (energy) and blood are like a never-ending, swift river, rushing on endlessly. An ancient saying maintains, "The moving water never will be putrid and the swinging door will not rot."

We should be most afraid of sluggish *qi* and blood circulation, since this slow movement allows the rapid growth of bacteria in localized areas. In the same way that slow-moving water will yield to bacteria and microorganisms and begin to smell, a person's body will become unafraid of growing bacteria and microorganisms, because the body houses these things to begin with. In other words, one's body might not recognize the invasion of malignant bacteria because it already houses similar bacteria. These bacteria can become an eruption, then a tumor, then a cancer, and will ultimately impair the heart's ability to pump and circulate the blood, resulting in illness and maybe even death.

Respiration

If there is no oxygen in your lungs, then there is no blood, according to Traditional Chinese Medicine (TCM). This premise is stated in *Huang Di Nei Jing* (The Inner Classic), a reference book used by TCM healers. The Inner Classic is said to have been written during the reign of the

Yellow Emperor, during the first and second century BC by the Yellow Emperor himself, probably with input from other authors. It is still studied today by all TCM practitioners as part of their training.

Anyway, The Inner Classic asserts that "*Qi* is the commander of the blood, and blood is the mother of the *qi*, and *qi* and blood support and depend upon each other."

Let me explain. The lungs dominate inhalation and exhalation. Inside the lungs there are *alveolis*—which are like sponges—soaking up blood containing carbon dioxide. When we inhale air, the carbon dioxide in the alveolis is exchanged with oxygen and the blood moves on. Therefore our blood has fresh oxygen.

Through the heart's main arteries the blood is transferred to the liver, and then enters the kidneys. The kidneys are like a filter. They store the essential materials, and discharge the toxic and harmful substances to the urinary bladder. The kidney stores *jing* (essence), responsible for reproduction, growth and development.

The ancient Chinese maintained that the kidney rules the bones, produces marrow; rules water; governs water metabolism, grasps lung *qi*; and receives *qi* from the lungs. Kidney *yang* controls "minister fire" (the pericardium, which protects the heart), activates spleen and lung, and is responsible for heart balance.

According to TCM, the kidneys are the foundation of the *yin and yang* (balance) of all the organs. The kidney is the gateway to the stomach, opens to the ears, manifests in the head hair, is responsible for hearing.

Circulation and Digestion

In the body, respiration is extremely important, but equally significant are the circulatory and digestive systems. These systems are closely related to the brain. The brain and the central nervous system cooperatively help each other. Without the nervous system there would be no reproductive and metabolic ability. The nervous system is connected to your entire body through your arteries, skin, muscles and tendons, and even reaches the hair on your head. The nerves can be in a state of *hypo-* (under) or *hyper-*(over) tension. These conditions contribute to the alteration of your bones.

For example, the lumbar nerves are connected to your muscles. If for some reason one side of the muscle is extremely tight, then the vertebra of your lower back will be bent and you will experience soreness and acute pain. Sometimes if you let your brain and mind relax; this allows your nerves to loosen up from the top to bottom. Even chronic lower back pain can be dissolved in this way.

This connection between your emotions and your physical body is an important component of your overall health situation. It is vital for individuals who have arthritis, or indeed anyone, to remember this basic philosophy of life: Live now! Don't worry about tomorrow, or even the next moment. Everyone has problems and situations in their life that they must deal with. There's no sense in burdening your mind and body with worry or fear about what might happen tomorrow, next week, or next year. Life is short. Enjoy each day, each moment. Enjoy your life. Be thankful and appreciate all that you have. Accept your limitations for what they are, carry on and do the best you can.

This poem, *Bringing in the Wine*, translated by Witter Bynner, describes this philosophy.

> See how the Yellow River's waters move out of heaven.
> Through silken-black at morning, have changed by night
> to snow.
> . . . Oh, let a man of spirit venture where he pleases
> And never tip his golden cup empty toward the moon!
> Since heaven gave the talent, let it be employed!
> Spin a thousand pieces of silver, all of them come back!

Cook a sheep, kill a cow, whet the appetite,
And make me, of three hundred bowls, one long drink!

* * *

The Chinese characters below say, *"Zhi Ji Zhi Bi, Bai Zhan Bai Shen."*

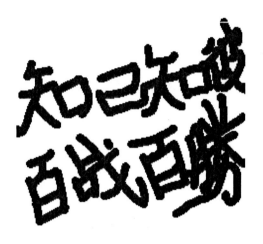

Zhi = Know, Understand
Ji = Self
Bi = Opponent
Bai = Hundred
Zhan = War
Shen = Win

The words, collectively, mean that you must understand yourself as well as your opponent so that you can win the war. We must approach arthritis with a similar attitude.

Chapter 2

Susan's Story

Before I go further into an explanation about what arthritis is, I'd like to share one patient's story with you.

Susan's Story

Susan came to see me, suffering a great deal from swollen knuckles, elbows that wouldn't straighten, sore wrists, shoulders and hips. Her feet hurt and her left knee was quite swollen. She was very pale, and looked and moved like an old woman. She was only 43 years old! Besides the pain from the swollen joints, she complained of fatigue, depression and weight loss, and was having trouble sleeping. She had suffered from acne and constipation for many years, and had ceased menstruating the previous year.

Susan said the symptoms started slowly, with a sore knee that would trouble her for a few days, and then get better. Then she started a new job, and noticed that she had trouble using a stapler and collating papers by hand. Again, it didn't seem any big deal, because it would get better when she didn't do those things.

It progressed, though, little by little, and soon she had trouble walking because her feet hurt. She began to lose strength in her hands, and had difficulty holding a pot when cooking dinner, or bending down to reach inside a low cupboard. She is an administrative assistant, and had always been able to type very quickly. Her fingers were so stiff that she couldn't keep up to her usual speed.

Susan had not been to a medical doctor, because she was afraid of facing what he had to say. She was fairly certain that she was suffering from arthritis, and she was scared that it was rheumatoid—the worst kind, her friends had told her. All her life her family had shied away from going to doctors unless absolutely necessary, preferring to cure ailments the "natural" way with herbs, vitamins and supplements. She had heard all kinds of horror stories about how debilitating arthritis would most certainly be, and did not want to admit she had it.

She had tried all sorts of health foods, supplements, and ointments, over the course of a year, and sometimes it seemed that the stiffness and swelling did get better. It always got bad again. She began to take ibuprofen daily, with little result. Her husband finally convinced her to come and see me. He works right next door to my clinic.

I could tell right away when I took her pulse that her blood was not good. Her left knee was swollen and puffy. She was very nervous and tense. I treated her with acupuncture, and asked her if she wanted to try some herbs. At the time she said no. After the treatment, she felt a little more relaxed.

I urged her to consult a medical doctor, and find out an exact diagnosis. She was afraid to go, but I assured her that finding out would only give us a starting point. She didn't need to be afraid of what she would find out—we could deal with anything.

She didn't put it off. Susan went to see the doctor the next day. She was told that she had all the textbook symptoms of rheumatoid arthritis, and that she would have to undergo treatment with drugs.

Maybe most people wouldn't have been upset by this news, but Susan was. Her family had always avoided taking any kind of drugs, even aspirin, unless absolutely necessary. Having to take "heavy duty" medication was not a popular option. The first doctor referred her to a rheumatologist.

The results of a blood test showed the rheumatologist that Susan's blood hemoglobin level was very low, her white blood cell count was high, and she was borderline anemic.

She spoke to her doctor about acupuncture and herbs, and decided that she would try a combination of western and eastern treatment.

Her doctor prescribed steroids plus an anti-inflammatory drug, the lowest level of medication that would both make Susan feel comfortable about taking it, and yet still relieve her symptoms. I prescribed tea made from Chinese herbs. She made the tea weekly, and drank three or four cups a day.

Susan's rheumatologist wanted to know what was in the herbs that I was giving her, and we provided her with a list. The doctor had no objection to Susan taking them.

Susan came to see me weekly, and I gave her a new "recipe" each time, depending on what her body's needs were. After awhile she was able to discontinue the steroid use, but she was still taking the anti-inflammatory medication prescribed by her rheumatologist, in addition to the Chinese herb tea. She also made and drank "bone soup." (See the recipe in a later chapter.)

After about two years on the medication, Susan began to develop bruising on her lower legs. The rheumatologist thought it could be caused by the Chinese herbs, and so asked Susan to stop drinking the tea. She did, for two months. Nothing changed. We thought we'd try a new tactic. We decided to try treating her more intensely with acupuncture and give her some herbs to balance her kidney yin. She stopped taking her prescription medication, and I began to treat her with acupuncture twice a week. I also encouraged her to drink more fluids on a daily basis.

After taking twice-weekly acupuncture treatments for about two months, and some three years after she first visited the rheumatologist, Susan is almost as flexible as she was before the onslaught of the disease. She has no more pain or joint swelling, is no longer constipated and has plenty of energy. She has gained back the weight she lost, and has put on an additional five pounds. The bruises are finally fading. She is thrilled to have regained her health, and at this time is continuing to use herbs to further strengthen her kidney and liver function.

Chapter 3

Why Did This Happen?

Why did this happen to me?

Usually, the answer to this question is an honest, "I don't know." Certainly there are some arthritic diseases, such as Lyme disease, with an obvious cause (infection by tick bite), but they are the minority. More often than not, modern medicine simply cannot explain why one person develops arthritis and another does not. However, we often have at least partial explanations.

People who have been recently diagnosed as having arthritis are usually full of questions. They want to know how their bodies are affected and what the future holds for their health. What does a joint look like? How does it change because of arthritis? What caused the disease in the first place? Is there a cure? What's the latest research?

Not all of the answers to these questions have been found, but researchers continue to find many promising leads. Scientists are well on their way to pinpointing causes of some of the major forms of arthritis, and they are also getting closer to finding drugs that will be able to stop the disease.

An important first step toward adjusting to arthritis is learning as much as possible about it. If you understand your chronic condition and the reasons behind your doctor's recommendations, you are more likely to adapt well. You learn why certain changes may occur and what to do about them. By seeking information, you choose to manage your health actively and not to be passively controlled by the disease.

You must also learn to handle the fear that often accompanies a diagnosis of arthritis. By learning as much as possible about your condition and your options, you take charge of your own health, and take a large step towards conquering your fears. Don't let fright control you. It can easily make your condition worse.

If you want to build a house you must first dig a hole. Then you pour in concrete to make a solid foundation. Without this solid foundation, the walls and floors that are built upon it are not sound and would topple easily. Therefore, in order to understand fully the concepts that follow, we must start with the basics—the foundation: the simplest definitions and principles.

What is a joint?

A joint is the place where the ends of two or more bones come together, usually in such a way that they can move. The bones in a joint are called articular bones. Bones and joints support our body (muscle, flesh, skin, and blood vessels), and can be called the body's frame. Joints are responsible for our body's movement, extension, flexion, circulation, and ability to carry items. Between the bones we have cartilage, and in order for us to have free and pleasant movement, some lubrication or fluid. In our bodies we have a total of 206 joints—in other words we have that many places that we need to protect, lubricate and nourish. All of these joints can become inflamed.

Anatomically, there are three types of joints: immobile joints, slightly moveable joints, and active, moveable joints.

Immobile joints

Synarthrodial joints are immobile joints. An example would be the skull. Not completely one bone, the skull is assembled from big and small bones—a whole bunch of different shapes joined together. Bone and bone connection areas look like gears, or butterfly wings. They are folded together very tightly at so-called suture joints, and sealed to protect the internal brain tissue.

Slightly moveable joints

Amphiarthrodial joints are slightly moveable joints. We often ignore these joints because they are only very slightly moveable. These joints are of special interest because many of them are not thought of as joints, yet they often become arthritic. The spine is an example of slightly moveable joints—a collection of bones called vertebral bodies, which are joined at facet joints. Human beings have seven cervical joints, 12 thoracic vertebrae, five lumbar vertebrae, plus the tailbone. All of these components can develop difficulty in their movement, even though they are only slightly moveable.

These slightly moveable joints can also cause referred pain elsewhere in the body. For example, what do we think when we have a sore heel? We believe that our shoes are the problem, or that we are walking too much. That backache you've attributed to muscle spasm could very well be arthritic in nature. We may believe that groin pain, or lower back pain, arises because of poor posture or walking position. How many of us understand that the pain may be the result of spinal problems?

The pelvis is another example of a collection of slightly moveable joints. The bones in the pelvis come together in the back at the sacroiliac joint, another joint that can become arthritic. There are a number of other slightly movable joints, many of which are the source of unsuspected arthritic pain.

Active moveable joints

Diarthrodial joints are freely moveable joints—the big joints that we are familiar with—such as the hip, elbow, knee and ankle. They can move easily and swing, allow big actions, and are characterized by fullness with strength. The bones joined by these joints bounce, extend, and contract. The ligaments joining them are just like rubber bands, and can be pulled long and twisted around the joint, connecting the bones with a lot of tissue to protect and connect.

Diarthrodial joints consist of a number of different structures. The first structure is an elastic material called cartilage, which is also present in some slightly movable joints. Cartilage provides a smooth surface that facilitates motion; thus, in most joints cartilage rubs against cartilage, not bone against bone. Ligaments hold the bones in a joint together, and tendons attach muscles to bones. The latter are similar to cables.

An *articular* capsule, the inside of which is lined by a material called *synovial* tissue or synovial membrane, surrounds all these structures. Synovial tissue produces antibodies, which protect the joint, as well as fluid, which bathes and lubricates the joint. Thus it is normal for joints to contain a small amount of fluid. The presence of excess fluid, however (water on the knee), is abnormal.

All types of joints, regardless of size and uniqueness to each other, have the same structure and ingredients and assembly. They all have cartilage, synovial membrane, and articular capsules. The only thing different is their shape, size, and location. In the clinic we see many kinds of arthritis and nerve and muscle aches that can exist in these slightly moveable and active moveable joints.

Bones

We've talked about what joints are, now let's talk a little about the composition of the bones that these joints connect. Bone forms the skeleton of the body. It is a reservoir of calcium, and acts as an anchor for

27

VALC

muscles, tendons and ligaments. Bone harbors many internal viscera including the central nervous system; it assists in the mechanism of respiration, and is a center of blood-forming activity and fat storage.

Bone contains an organic protein matrix seeded with inorganic
minerals—mostly calcium and magnesium salts. On average by weight,
bone is 65% mineral, and 35% organic tissue. These elements and
bone's concentric tubular structure provide both strength and flexibility. There is a slight amount of water in bone, with calcium making up about two-thirds of its composition and phosphorous the remaining one-third. The phosphorous makes bone pliant while calcium makes it hard and brittle.

Bone tissue can be compact or *cancellous*. Compact bone (also called
cortical bone) contains channels holding blood vessels and nerves that
supply nutrients and remove waste. Cancellous bone tissue is of spongy, or
porous structure.

Most of us don't realize that all bones are continuously, actively me-
tabolizing and being replaced. It does not matter whether they are big
bones with big joints or small bones with small joints—their internal
structures are the same.

What is Arthritis?

Derived from the Greek, meaning "inflammation of a joint," arthritis
is an inflammation classically consisting of redness, pain, heat, and swelling. The term is often confusing, however, because all four of these elements may not appear together.

According to the estimate of scientists, roughly 97% of human beings
have arthritis or osteoarthritis. I say we all have some illness in our joints
unless we are not using them, such as in the case of a newborn baby, or a
person who is in a coma.

According to modern medicine the cause of arthritis is unknown. Osteoarthritis appears to be due to a complex of interacting mechanical, biological, biochemical, and enzymatic feedback loops. When one or more of these components fails to do its job properly, this sets in motion the changes in the joint tissue that we call arthritis.

Some factors that may contribute to the onset of arthritis are congenital joint abnormalities, genetic defects, infections, metabolic, endocrine, and neuropathic diseases. Neuropathic diseases are virtually any diseases that alter the normal structure and function of the cartilage covering the inner surfaces of the joint, and acute and chronic trauma affecting this cartilage. In terms of this last cause, we are talking about wear and tear.

Truthfully, the how, why, and what happens in arthritis are still unknown. We can guess that it may be related to your heritage, happen as a result of old injuries, because of degeneration of bones, from your metabolism losing balance, from infection or inflammation and may even be deeply related to your job, lifestyle, and diet.

Generally speaking, in my view, there are five kinds of arthritis, which can be divided by pathology or physiology. What I mean by pathology is a disease, something you can prevent. Physiology means something kind of normal, like what happens to our bodies as we age. However, it does not matter what kind of arthritis we have, whether its cause is pathology or physiology, since both cause problems when we try to move our joints. The result is the same—it is painful and inconvenient.

The five kinds of arthritis are:

1. Osteoporosis arthritis. What usually happens in old age, and involves thinning bone density and joint breakdown.
2. Osteoarthritis. The chronic breakdown of cartilage in the joints.
3. Rheumatoid arthritis. An autoimmune form of arthritis, which causes inflammation in the lining of the joints and/or other internal organs.
4. Rheumatic arthritis. Caused by bacterial infection.

5.   Traumatized arthritis. Can appear at the site of a previous injury.

Briefly, osteoporosis is caused by a hormone imbalance, which causes the bones to degenerate. The next three types have to do with our heritage, our DNA, or our diet. The fifth type, traumatized arthritis, can occur in a previously injured joint.

Chapter 4

Causes, Signs, Symptoms

What causes disease?

In the western or modern medical point of view, pain or distress, injury, harm, life-threatening disease or even death, generally speaking, can happen to the body in two ways, through physiological or pathological means.

Physiology is the branch of biology that deals with the functions of living organisms and their components. It basically describes life processes in terms of physics and chemistry. Anatomy is the structural counterpart and, in a historical sense, the parent of physiology. Physiology deals with a procedure or deviation from a normal condition—such as birth, growth, aging, and to cease living. Physiology has to do with the natural functional way of life.

On the other hand, pathology is the branch of medicine that deals with the causes and processes of disease and its effects on the structure and function of the human body. All physicians are involved to some extent in pathology, but a pathologist specializes in interpreting processes of disease by examination of tissues and body fluids obtained during surgery or autopsy.

Simply stated, pathology is the scientific study of disease and its causes from an outside factor, such as a plant, animal, bacterium, unicellular organism, fungus, slime mold, and certain algae. All of these poisonous substances are produced by living cells or organisms and are capable of causing disease when introduced into the body. The consequent development of disease that may threaten life is called pathology.

The TCM view of disease is different. Chinese medical professionals believe and accept that disease is caused by other factors, especially the following:

Irregular food intake.

What is irregular eating? According to eastern practitioners, it includes eating too little or too much, eating raw or cold foods, greasy foods, hot spicy foods, eating too fast or fasting, eating irregular amounts. Any eating pattern that is out of the usual in this context means irregular food intake. The consequence will induce indigestion, impaired digestion or "upset stomach" and disorder of the stomach.

Here's an example. A member of a local military unit wants to harass and undermine the enemy. The best method is by surprise—attacking when and where the enemy least expects it. In the case of the human body, the outside forces can get the best results by attacking the stomach in an unexpected manner. Of course it is not good for the stomach!

The Inner Classic says the stomach is the sea of nourishment, of water and grain, in the upper abdomen. The stomach governs the decomposition of food. The stomach and spleen are the root of post-natal qi. What on earth am I saying? Basically, what I mean is the actions of stomach and spleen together form the foundation of the body's energy.

Sexual Overactivity.

Excessive sexual activity is not only physical work and strains the muscles, but also depletes kidney jing. We know the kidney stores kidney jing (essence), is responsible for reproduction, growth and development, rules the bones, produces marrow, rules water, governs water metabolism, grasps lung *qi*, and receives *qi* from the lungs.

Kidney *yang* controls "minister fire" (the pericardium), activates spleen and lung, is responsible for heart balance. Kidneys are the foundation of *the yin and yang* of all the organs. They are the gateway to the stomach, open to the ears, manifest in the head hair, are responsible for hearing. Sexual overactivity can deplete the kidney's reserves of *jing*, affecting all of these areas. Even early marriage or excessive birthing can damage kidney essence and lead to a deficient and weak body, low backaches, pains and soreness.

For females, excessive birthing will damage the *chong/ren* meridian. In TCM we believe the *chong/ren* meridian function is as follows:

Ren meridian (Conception Vessel, or Directing Channel):
   Governor of the *yin* meridian or sea of *yin* meridian.
   Closely related to infertility and menstruation.

Chong meridian (Penetrating Channel, or Thrusting Channel):
   Sea of 5 *Zang*/6 *Fu* (Day / Night organs)
   Sea of 12 regular meridians
   Sea of Blood

Damage to the *chong/ren* meridian function can result in irregular menstruation, *amenorrhea* or *leukorrhea*.

Physical Overexertion.

Excessive physical work, for example, too much lifting, affects the lower back, kidney and groin area. Four fingers below the umbilicus is the *"dantien,"* what the Chinese medical practitioner calls the "source" of *qi*. In this example, a person who lifts and moves boxes or equipment uses his abdomen and low back. He complains of soreness and tiredness. Without proper rest, his source of *qi*, and thus the kidney, become weak, affecting the entire body. Overexertion can sometimes also lead to injury of the spleen, and a lowered immune system function as well.

Qi Kong masters teach people to breathe all the way down to and from the dantien, the source of *qi*. The body strengthens and nourishes the *dantien* in this way.

Other Causes of Disease.

Trauma (damaged skin, flesh, tendon, bone, *qi*/blood)

Burns (fire or chemical/acid burn)

Snake bite, insect bite (i.e. mosquito)

Mucus (mainly due to loss of balance in the metabo-lism of lung, kidney, spleen, and internal organs)

Result of normal physiology (i.e., six pathogenic fac-tors—more about this in Chapter 6)

Over-secretion of bodily liquids

Blood stagnation, representing

1) The whole body's blood circulation obstruction;

2) Local blood stagnation; and/or

3) Blood running out of meridians and retained in certain areas (sometimes occurs in *Zang Fu* tissue organs and vessels).

According to TCM, these are the main conditions that cause disease in the body. Later on I'll explain more about the six pathogenic factors: wind, cold, dampness, heat, dryness and fire, and how they relate to disease. Right now, though, let's get back to our main subject, and talk about the characterization of arthritis.

Signs & Symptoms of Clinical Arthritis

Arthritis is classified as a painful syndrome, or bi syndrome, according to The Inner Classic (*Huang Di Nei Jing*), a reference book familiar to all Traditional Chinese medicine practitioners. Arthritis is greatly related to diet, living habits, and environment. Painful syndromes are mainly characterized by pain, soreness, numbness and heaviness of the muscles and joints with limitation of movement. However, the form of pain may vary from patient to patient: very severe pain usually suggests intense causative factors or severe *qi* and blood stagnation.

In a machine, lubricated bearings are supposed to reduce the noise and rubbing as it works. However, when the bearings become rusted, the machine loses its normal function. It starts to make noises and its parts may warp or break down. When our human body's bearings become rusted from lack of lubrication, our bones and joints may begin to deteriorate. We will feel pain, experience limited motion, and sometimes hear cracking or grating sounds when we move.

Since there are different signs and symptoms for arthritis, there are different names for each type, including Osteoarthritis, Rheumatoid Arthritis, Systemic Lupus Erythematosus, Scleroderma, Polymyositis and Dermatomyositis, Ankylosing Spondylitis, Reiter's Syndrome, Gout, Pseudo Gout, Infectious Arthritis, Psoriatic Arthritis, Polymyalgia Rheumatic and Giant Cell Arthritis, Fibrositis, Bursitis, etc. In my experience there are five kinds of arthritis, and all of these listed above are only different names or versions of these five types.

1. Osteoporosis Arthritis (Bone Mass Loss Arthritis)

Osteoporosis arthritis and osteoarthritis, which we will talk about next, are not the same. A recent survey indicates that many American women confuse osteoporosis with osteoarthritis.

Osteoporosis is a condition in which the bones and joints deteriorate and break down. It is a preventable and treatable affliction, often called a "silent" disease because it can progress for years without symptoms before a fracture occurs.

Contrary to what many people believe, bone is living tissue. Throughout life, bone tissue constantly breaks down and is replaced by new bone tissue. As we age, and particularly after women reach menopause, bones tend to break down more quickly than they can rebuild. Osteoporosis occurs when not enough new bone is formed or when too much of the calcium or other components are lost (or both). The bones become thin and prone to fracture. Why does this happen?

Some people call bone mass loss arthritis the combination menopause syndrome. It starts from endocrine imbalance, which makes the bones' *osteoblast* and *osteoclast* cells miscalculate, causing bone mass to flow away. Bones become porous, fragile, easily cracked, and lose calcium. The space between bones may increase or the bones themselves may warp.

According to scientists, our brains give a signal to stimulate the secretion of our hormone estrogen. This hormone decides how much marrow and nutrition we should store in our bones. When a woman reaches the cycle of menopause, production of estrogen is reduced. The estrogen signal that used to be sent to the ovary to begin menstruation is no longer sent, and no menses occur. The woman's body can become confused and out of balance because of the lack of this hormone. The body's osteoblasts and osteoclasts are not able to calculate the amount of marrow remaining in the bones, or how much marrow and calcium or other materials to produce.

Don't feel too sad if you are a woman, men begin to suffer from osteoporosis as well, only a little bit later – around age 65.

If a person doesn't know this whole theory, or understand this process, he or she doesn't know to take in more nutrients and try to slow down this bone loss crisis.

Another example where osteoporosis might occur is in a person who has suffered from a stroke. Because he is not able to walk by himself and likes to lie down all the time, the man's bones will become very brittle and easily broken. Why are his bones so weak? As a person ages, his bones do not rebuild as they did when he was younger. A great deal of nutritional intake is needed to encourage bone and marrow re-growth. Exercise is also very important in the formation of bone, and lack of it can contribute to osteoporosis.

2. Osteoarthritis

Osteoarthritis is a painful degenerative joint disease that results in a reduction of mobility and function. When most people talk about arthritis, they are talking about osteoarthritis. Osteoarthritis is diagnosed on the basis of its symptoms and on can be seen on x-rays. It is possible to have both osteoarthritis and osteoporosis at the same time, although people who have osteoarthritis seem to have a lower risk of developing osteoporosis.

Osteoarthritis is a chronic disease that involves breakdown of the joint tissue, primarily the cartilage. It is perhaps the oldest and most common disease of humans and goes by a variety of other names, including degenerative joint disease, osteoarthrosis, and hypertrophic arthritis. Probably every person past age 60 has osteoarthritis to some degree, but only a minority have it badly enough to notice any symptoms. Sometimes, however, they feel pain, experience limited motion, and require medical care.

Osteoarthritis affects only the joints and surrounding tissues. In a healthy joint, the tissues are flexible and elastic, and movement is easy. The first major change in a joint affected with osteoarthritis is that the smooth cartilage surface softens and becomes pitted and frayed. The cartilage loses its elasticity and is more easily damaged by stress. At first, the degraded cartilage cells are replaced, but this repair process eventually begins to fail. With time, large sections of cartilage may be worn away completely, leaving the ends of the bones unprotected. Without their normal gliding surfaces, joint movement becomes painful.

As the cartilage continues to break down, the joint loses its normal shape and mechanical structure. The bone ends thicken due to abnormal growth of cartilage and bone and form "spurs" of bone called osteophytes at the points where the ligaments and joint capsule attach to the bone. The ligaments may also thicken. Fluid-filled sacs sometimes form in the bone near the joint, and bits of bone or cartilage called "joint mice" may float loosely in the joint space, contributing to the pain that occurs with movement. As a rule, only a moderate amount of inflammation occurs and is probably the result of loose pieces of bone and cartilage irritating the joint lining *(synovium)*.

There are two categories of osteoarthritis: primary and secondary. Primary osteoarthritis appears without any obvious cause. Secondary osteoarthritis develops in joints that have previously sustained damaging injuries.

An example of secondary osteoarthritis is the condition called "baseball finger" in which a ball repeatedly hits a fingertip. The injury later leads to the development of osteoarthritis in the finger joint. This may also occur in joints affected by infections, previous fractures, or by another type of arthritis such as rheumatoid arthritis. Sometimes, years of supporting extra weight (obesity) leads to secondary osteoarthritis in the weight-bearing joints.

3. Rheumatoid Arthritis

Rheumatoid arthritis is an *autoimmune* disease in which the body attacks its own healthy tissues. Autoimmune diseases are a result of immune systems that are too strong or too weak.

The body's white cells, or *leukocytes*, are involved in the immune system's ability to distinguish normal cells from foreign invaders. A popular theory among arthritis experts is that some people's immune systems respond abnormally to infections, resulting in chronic inflammation. The white blood cells of the immune system move from the bloodstream into the joint tissues. The membrane surrounding the joints becomes inflamed and releases enzymes that can cause the surrounding cartilage and bone to deteriorate.

Anyone can get rheumatoid arthritis, although it usually occurs in the young to middle adult years, and is more common in women. Occasionally people with rheumatoid arthritis will develop inflammation of the membranes surrounding the heart and lungs. They may also develop dry eyes and a dry mouth due to inflammation of tear glands and salivary glands.

4. Rheumatic Arthritis

Rheumatic arthritis is caused by bacterial infection. Sometimes it can lead to bone, joint, and muscle disease—even heart disease. In severe cases, inflammation and infection can cause heart failure, rheumatic heart disease, and loss of life.

Generally rheumatic arthritis is caused by outside sources, a bacterial infection from the likes of streptococcus, staphylococcus or gonorrhea, that is transferred to joints. In the clinic we can see symptoms of redness, heat, swelling, and pain.

Rheumatic arthritis can happen anywhere in the body, however it appears most often in the wrist, knee and elbow. It is always accompanied by fever—sometimes a high fever.

People with rheumatic arthritis should seek immediate medical attention because the bacterial infection in the joints will eventually cripple them. If rheumatic arthritis spreads to the heart valves, it can cause death.

5. Traumatized arthritis

Trauma, sports injury or overuse of muscles and joints can result in traumatized arthritis. For example, if we have not taken proper care of the ligaments, muscles, and tendons, bones and joints in the wrist and have continuously overused them, the result can be a "natural" traumatized joint.

Unnatural trauma, caused by outside forces such as falls, sprains, car accidents, etc., could become a future site for traumatized arthritis. Although we have taken care of the trauma medically, for example, set the broken ankle, it may not have completely healed.

Traumatized arthritis can stem from a group of muscles that have been injured or chronically abused. When the body attempts to repair the injury, it tries to produce more bone and marrow. Because of this excess of bone and marrow, joint *synovial* fluid loosens and increases in thickness. Ligaments also increase in thickness and put pressure on the root of nerves. The abuse can also cause blood circulation problems.

The clinical signs and symptoms of traumatized arthritis are local pain, joint cracking sounds, limited mobility or lack of mobility. The joint itself will have excess fluid retention. Around the joint there will be an excess of bone growth, or bone spurs, and the space between the bones will become very narrow. In the later stages of traumatized arthritis, the joint will become irregularly shaped, the surface will become marred with different grooves and movement will be very painful.

Regardless of the type of arthritis you have, in order to retain or regain normal joint movement, you must find an individual treatment that considers all the factors that pertain to your life and your body.

In the Eastern point of view, there are two types of arthritis, which are called syndromes: *wei* and *bi* syndrome. Both *wei* and *bi* cause weakness in your limbs, making it difficult to exercise, causing numbness in your four limbs, pain and spasms. However, upon closer examination, *wei* and bi are different from each other.

Wei syndrome occurs when your internal heat damages your blood vessels. The heat that causes this generally comes from your lungs or your stomach. Excess heat from the stomach could move upwards and burn your lungs, or sometimes it could be your lungs that are producing their own heat.

According to the Five-Element Theory, another of the important eastern medical theories, the lung belongs to metal, opens into your nose and manifests in your skin. Metal must be clear and shining—this way the *qi* in your body will be able to circulate. However, if this metal is not shiny or clear, *wei* syndrome may manifest. *Wei* syndrome means that muscles and/or tendons have atrophied. Modern medicine says that *wei* is a neuritis problem, possibly caused by the effects of polio that has not been fully cured. There is restricted mobility and little range of motion.

In the ancient Chinese book Yellow Emperor, better known as the "Inner Classic," there is a phrase that says, *"Fei Re Yeh Jiao,"* which translates to Burnt Leaves Caused by Heated Tree. The ancient Chinese believed that your lungs were like a canopy or tree, and when they became overheated your bronchi, or leaves, would become burnt. Once the bronchi burn they cannot nourish your organs, skin and tendons. This causes the undernourished organ to function incorrectly or not at all.

The way to correct this undernourishment is to bring one's digestion

41

back to normal, thus ending the *wei* syndrome. *Wei* syndrome is divided into five different categories:

1. Skin. When your skin has *wei* syndrome, its color is lackluster. Hair follicles begin to fall out and you will begin to find that you are short of breath.

2. Muscle. In the case of muscle *wei* syndrome, your skin begins to take on a yellow shade and the muscle feels like an overripe peach. Usually this has to do with heat in your spleen.

3. Tendon *wei* causes your skin to become pale and gives you a bitter taste in your mouth. Your nails lack luster and your tendons will spasm. This usually is because of the excess heat in your liver.

4. Meridian *wei* causes your skin to become reddish in color, caused by the heat in your heart.

5. Bone *wei* causes your skin to darken and your ears look like they have been burned. Your waist and knee become sore, usually caused by excess heat in your kidneys.

These five types of *wei* are all caused by excess heat. The excess heat in the body is caused by an accumulation of damp heat, damp mucus, qi deficiency, blood deficiency, yin deficiency, blood stagnation, and/or food stagnation. These problems happen because your ascending and descending pathways, or meridians, are obstructed. Please bear with me—I will explain more about all these theories in a later chapter.

Bi syndrome is more like the Western medical definition of arthritis.

> If he has bone *bi* the person will feel that his limbs are very heavy and uncomfortable when lifting.

> In meridian *bi* the blood stagnates and cannot circulate.

In tendon *bi*, extending the limb is difficult but retracting is easy.

In muscle *bi* the four limbs are difficult to use.

In skin *bi* the skin loses its sensitivity.

When *bi* meets coldness, the whole body tightens.

When *bi* meets heat, the body becomes flaccid.

A person with *bi* becomes irritable, will sometimes pant, will become nauseated. This is because *bi* stays in the lung as a guest. Irritability is from rebellion of qi in the chest.

When *bi* is a guest in the heart, one will have symptoms of throat dryness, and become easily startled. The body will feel cold and swollen, and the abdomen will feel full.

Extreme thirst, frequent urination, a feeling of fullness in the area below the belly button, and easily wakening from sleep for no reason are all causes of *bi* being a guest in the liver.

When a patient's limbs become swollen easily, and he feels tension in his bladder, bowels, eyes, ears, nose, and throat, this means that *bi* is a guest in the kidney. The person hunches over and his nine orifices feel swollen.

You can determine that *bi* is a guest in the spleen when a patient's four limbs are tired and lazy, he coughs and vomits with a little bit of phlegm. Sometimes the person will feel like something is stuck in his upper trachea.

Clinically *wei* and *bi* both cause difficulty in range of motion. They both cause the person to become very thin and seem sickly. Generally speaking, the difference between *wei* and *bi* syndrome is whether there is pain or lack of pain. *Wei* syndrome causes tendons and meridians to become flaccid and soft. Those afflicted with *wei* syndrome become weak, and are not able to exercise, but there is no pain—only weakness. *Bi* syndrome, however, causes both pain and weakness. The tendons and muscles are very tight with much chronic pain.

According to the above we can come to two conclusions: *Wei* syndrome relates to excess, and *bi* relates to deficiency.

Deficiency means that the spleen, stomach, liver and kidney functions are all inadequate. Excess means that there is obstruction or stagnation due to dampness and heat. A further complication may be lung heat, which injures the body fluids. This problem is caused by excess combined with deficiency, therefore diagnosis must be made with extreme care. If it is *wei* syndrome, acupuncture, massage, and physical therapy are all good methods of treatment. Either way, if the diagnosis is *bi* or *wei*, early prevention and treatment leads to a better prognosis.

The characters below represent *Bi* syndrome:

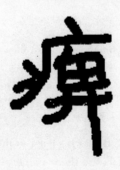

Bi Syndrome
"Tong Zhe Bu Tong, Tong Zhe Bu Tong"
Tong= Through
Zhe= Then
Bu= No

Tong = Painful. In certain cases, the Chinese language dictates that you must emphasize his word, thus changing it's meaning.

The meaning of *Bi* Syndrome according to this statement is: If you are suffering from pain, then it means you are suffering from obstruction. No obstruction, no pain.

TCM philosophy dictates that because your body system is not clean, it causes you pain. If everything in your body system is clear and free of obstruction, there will be no more pain or blockage.

Imagine that your house is filled with all sorts of garbage. What would you do? Would you, like many other people, stuff it all into trash bags and take it out to the dumpster? And would that be the end of the story?

Continue to imagine that you throw all of your junk down the sink. Sooner or later your drain will clog and any running water will back up. Similarly, we all know what problems come with driving a high mileage car. Since its engine has been overused, its cylinders and pistons have been scraped against each other, causing deformity and bringing mechanical deterioration, thus wasting fuel. The fuel cannot be completely used and cannot evaporate, thereby forming a solid substance that blocks proper engine function.

In order to bring the engine back to proper function, we must clear the blockage and add fluids to allow free movement of the engine's parts. To restore the arthritic body to proper function, we must clear the blockages, allow free circulation of blood and other fluids, and assimilate nutrition.

Chapter 5

Self Diagnosis

Trying to diagnose oneself sounds like a very difficult process. You might say, "I'm not a doctor. I don't have a medical background, I'm not trained for it and I don't know how to diagnose."

How about if I told you that self-diagnosis is very easy? If you follow the procedure step by step you'll be able to diagnose yourself—or at least you'll know your problem clearly.

As we know, every time we have a problem and we go to see our medical doctor, he or she will ask a whole bunch of questions and then, if necessary, they'll take some blood or urine and send it to the lab. Then they'll give us a diagnosis.

But do you know that when the doctor starts to ask questions, he is collecting information from us? We call it signs. So the patient gives to him the signs. And then the doctor collects these signs and determines what kind of syndrome they fit. He combines these signs and syndromes, and together, they make a pattern. This we call pattern recognition.

The doctor examines this pattern and matches it to some kind of terminology—what we call diagnosis. If he is not sure he'll ask for blood or urine samples to send to the lab to be studied. The results will give the physician enough information to help him make a diagnosis. And that's the way it is. What's most important is the information that the patient gives to the doctor.

So you understand that we have to give the doctor the signs or complaints or tell him what's wrong with us. The complaints, or chief complaint, are what the patient explains to the doctor as being the most bothersome problem. So if we know how to complain, then we know how to diagnose, at least in the western point of view.

However, on the eastern side, complaining is viewed as more than that. To an eastern practitioner, diagnosis means trying to find out the underlying reason for what's wrong. More important is the difference between diagnosis A and diagnosis B, called differentiation. Equally important to the eastern physician is what is causing A to do this and what is causing B to do that. This is called differentiation as well.

When we know what the difference is between this syndrome and that syndrome, then we can treat the problem. We treat the problem from the root as well as the branches, which represent the present condition. The present condition is the main component of the case, including the onset, development, diagnosis and treatment of the disease. Understanding the present disease is helpful for the doctor to analyze the affliction, find its development patterns and get the basics for establishing diagnosis.

How to Analyze the Disease

1. **The onset.** This refers to the time taken to induce the cause and mode of onset—sudden or gradual. In other words, have you been suffering with the symptoms for a long time, steadily getting worse, or did it happen suddenly?

   Understanding the onset factors will help predict the deficiency or excess (cold or heat) of the disease. For example, if the disease attacks suddenly and lasts for a short time, it pertains to excess syndrome. If the disease comes on slowly and exists for a long time, the pattern pertains to deficiency syndrome.

2. **The characteristics of the main symptoms.** This includes symptom location, nature and duration. To get some idea of these characteristics it is helpful in judging the location and the nature of pathological change. For instance, if the main symptoms are characterized by dull pain in the abdomen that may be relieved by warmth and pressure, this suggests insufficiency of spleen *yang*. Soreness and weakness in the loins and knees, intolerance of coldness and cold extremes manufactures deficiency of kidney *yang*.

Maybe you're still confused. Let me make a long story short. Just simply answer for yourself such questions as, "How does this disease work?" "How did it develop?" "What is the treatment process?" "Is the present disease related to some other disease?" "Do my family members—relatives, parents—have this problem as well?" "Is it related to my lifestyle, diet?" "Do I over stress?" "Is it related to my working condition?" "Is it related to my living space/climate?"

"Is there any syndrome besides the chief complaint?" You might call this a secondary syndrome. This refers to other syndromes accompanying the main one. Understanding their characteristics is significant to the differentiation between excess and deficiency (cold and heat) of the disease.

Here's an example. If the patient's main symptom is insomnia, which is accompanied by palpitation, irritability, red tongue with little coating, thready and rapid pulse, this may be considered as the syndrome heart *yin* disease. When accompanied by a tendency to become frightened, bitter taste in the mouth, yellowish and greasy tongue coating, slippery and rapid pulse, it should be regarded as a syndrome of gall bladder stagnation with disturbance of phlegm.

After we make our first self-diagnosis, every now and then we should re-examine ourselves. How was this diagnosis made, what medicine or treatment has been taken and how effective is the medicine? Re-diagnose your current situation.

When you re-diagnose yourself you should keep in mind the following points:

> Cold and heat are usually associated with the nature of the disease, and with the excess or deficiency of *yin* or *yang* in the body.
> Diseases due to affliction of pathogenic cold usually show cold signs.
> Diseases due to attack of pathogenic heat often manifest as heat signs.
> Excess of *yin*, or deficiency of *yang*, appear as a cold syndrome in most cases.
> Excess of *yang*, or deficiency of *yin*, appear as a heat syndrome in most cases.

Therefore to ask yourself whether you feel cold or feverish may help not only in learning the nature of the disease, but also in judging if there is an excess or deficiency in *yin* or *yang*. The syndromes due to pathogenic cold or heat appear clinically as follows:

Cold Syndrome

If you cannot endure cold and you find no relief by adding heat, the cause is often found in exterior syndrome produced by an outside source. This pathogen could be a virus, bacteria, or other microorganism that invades the exterior of the body, causing *yang* obstruction or deficiency. When *yang* is obstructed or deficient, the structure and musculature fail to warm. In other words, in exterior syndrome, your body is under attack by an external disease-producing agent.

If you cannot stand cold, but are able to get relief by adding exterior

49

warmth, this is usually due to miscellaneous disease because of internal injuries. The *yang* qi (energy) is insufficient and the structure and musculature cannot be warmed.

Heat syndrome

Fever in TCM is considered to be present when the patient's temperature is higher than normal, or also when his temperature is normal, but he feels feverish. If fever and aversion to cold occur simultaneously, the cause is usually due to an exterior syndrome affected by outside factors. If the patient feels feverish but is not averse to cold, the case is often a syndrome of internal heat.

Differentiating between cold syndrome and heat syndrome is very important to the eastern practitioner in determining the method of treatment for each person's situation.

Chapter 6

Medication Side-Effects

What are my treatment options?

At present, Western medical treatment for all kinds of arthritis is usually in the form of medication. To the big eared, tiny human being (I call us this because much of what we do depends on what we hear), who one day happens to have the agony and torture of joint pain, the simplest solution is to ease the pain.

Because that tiny joint is painful, it is not practical to let it influence a man's job too much because he has children, a wife, a mortgage and bills to pay, or some other type of headache that needs to be taken care of. Therefore, there is no time to worry about joint pain. The man runs directly to the pharmacy to buy big bottles, small bottles—whatever he can get his hands on—and pours a whole bunch of pills into his mouth, hoping that the pain will stop. Sometimes it does. Sometimes several hours later the pain will resume and the person will do the same thing again.

This is what nine out of ten people do. We try all sorts of over-the-counter painkillers, and if one brand doesn't work, we try another.

What do you know about painkillers?

Acetaminophen and *nonsteroidal anti-inflammatory drugs (NSAIDS)* are both are called painkillers, but what are the differences?

Acetaminophen, of the so-called *para-aminophenols*—well known as *Tylenol, Datril*, and *Liquiprin*—generally speaking only takes care of fever and pain. Acetaminophen is an analgesic, which reduces or eliminates pain, and an antipyretic, which reduces fever. Common side effects of acetaminophen are gastrointestinal symptoms, liver toxicity, and renal complications.

Non-steroidal anti-inflammatory drugs are often called *NSAIDS*, (pronounced n-sayds) or *salicylates, acetic acid, propionic acid, fenamic acid*, or *oxicans*. They all fight pain, lower fever and reduce inflammation, so the difference between acetaminophen and NSAIDS is that NSAIDS have ingredients to control inflammation.

Common side effects of salicylates, or NSAIDS, are:

> Disturbed digestion or indigestion, epigastric pain, flatulence, nausea, vomiting, cramps.
>
> Renal symptoms such as renal hypertension—arterial disease in which chronic high blood pressure is the primary symptom—toxicity in the urine, or toxicity of the kidneys' condition. *Oliguria* may occur, which is insufficient urine, or renal failure, which is no excretion of urine.
>
> Bleeding disorders.
>
> Hypersensitivity, which shows up in skin rash, itching, or *anaphylacis*, a generally temporary severe physical or emotional trauma.
>
> A severe reaction could include marked loss of blood pressure and depression of vital processes, or shock.

There are more than 20 over-the-counter painkillers in common use in the United States, including aspirin, *Tylenol, Advil, Motrin, Naprosyn*,

Aleve, Orudis, and *Feldene.* Some of these drugs are classed as anti-inflammatory, and are often used for the pain of arthritis. However, some researchers agree that while pharmaceutical companies continue to produce new versions of the same thing—anti-inflammatory drugs to reduce the pain of osteoarthritis—the disease tends to be mostly non-inflammatory. In the later stages of osteoarthritis you might occasionally find inflammation present.

Also, there is some preliminary evidence that anti-inflammatories obstruct the ability of cartilage cells to heal. So all you're doing when you take an anti-inflammatory is covering up the pain, and probably impairing the healing process at the same time. Covering up the pain does not address the cause, and may in fact worsen it.

Many people take acetaminophen to stop pain and reduce fever. In ancient times, humans would take willow tree bark and extract its sap and drink it in order to reduce nerve pain, headache, muscle aches and joint pain. Now we have synthetic willow bark sap, with a new name, "aspirin." We use aspirin and other similar products such as Tylenol, Anacin-3, Nuprin and Panadol. Some of them can reduce the pain, temporarily.

However, all these painkillers or pharmaceuticals leave something behind, which we call side effects. These drugs are unnatural substances chemically created to mimic the effects of the natural remedy. They are foreign to the body, but their components are often too infinitesimal for the body to recognize them. These particles get past the immune system's safeguards, and since the body doesn't know what to do with them, they settle in various organs or systems.

Side effects of these types of painkillers are usually, first of all, gastrointestinal interference. Stomach and intestines feel uncomfortable, there is a loss of appetite, and the individual becomes hungry but has no desire to eat. (If the person forces himself to eat, he feels nauseous and often wants to vomit what's just been eaten.) There may be burning sensations in the chest, and in severe cases, stomach bleeding or ulcers. Normal stomach function is damaged.

Some scientific reports have indicated that long term use of aspirin will create a high frequency noise in the ear, also called *tinnitus*. In severe cases it even causes loss of balance while moving or walking, and the feeling of not being able to walk in a straight line. In my clinical experience, I have found another side effect of aspirin to be that the blood-clotting time in a patient using aspirin is longer than that of a non-aspirin user.

When an acupuncture needle is inserted into the same point in two patients, one who is on pain-relievers, the other who is not, different results are noticed when it is time to withdraw the needle. Normally, you put pressure on the needle hole with a cotton ball for one to two minutes, and the bleeding stops. However, the chronic pain-relief user will need around five minutes before the blood clots. Sometimes bleeding will stop for a while, and then resume. This is because the amount of platelets in the blood is decreased, causing the blood to be less dense.

In the long run, the chronic painkiller-user's liver function is reduced. The liver becomes thicker, sometimes develops inflammation, and begins to erode. We all know that the liver is like a large chemical factory. It produces a large amount of chemical elements for the body's needs. When the chemical elements are insufficient, the physical body will undergo strange reactions, such as spasms, headaches, dizziness, blurred vision and other types of unusual behavior. Also, the liver produces bile. When the liver's ability to function is insufficient it will indirectly influence the gall bladder's bile secretion. Therefore the gall bladder system will also be damaged.

In the clinic, you will see the painkiller-user overreacting, over-exaggerating, oversensitive. He is very picky about his food intake. If food is not eaten with care, he will feel bloated, constipated, nauseous, uncomfortable in the stomach, and have low energy and weakness in the body.

The overuse of painkillers will also eventually cause serious problems in the kidneys.

We are all aware that every person has a pair of kidneys. The kidneys' main mission is to filter impurities from the blood. The kidneys keep the individual's water, urine and alkaline level balanced at a certain pH.

If the kidneys lose their normal function, then blood pressure will rise. Just think about a water hose: if you hold down a certain part, the water coming out will become a thin stream with very high pressure. Keeping that in mind, supporting the blood's circulation is the heart. If there is an obstruction, the heart needs to use quite a bit of strength to push through it. This is the particular moment when cerebral accidents occur—stroke, shock, bleeding, or what we call in TCM *windstroke*. Windstroke can be called cerebral hemorrhage, cerebral thrombosis, cerebral embolism, or apoplexy. The onset of the event is acute—it happens with great speed, like the wind blowing. This is why we call it windstroke.

Because the kidneys are not providing the usual safeguards, they can become inflamed from infection. Every time you have inflammation in your kidneys, your body must send many white cells there to help fight the infection. Sometimes these extra white cells can obstruct the kidney tubes, causing increased uric acid, its residue or other garbage to remain in the kidney, not able to be expelled. Acid poisoning can result, which in severe cases causes death. In some mild cases acid poisoning will damage the kidneys or cause urinary tract obstruction, kidney stones, and/or hardening of the arteries. In the clinic we will see these effects manifest as edema, usually in the foot and ankle. (Usually in the afternoon when we are out of energy, the edema is worse).

All pharmaceuticals can create unpredictable results. No one's body reacts in exactly the same way as another. Other side effects caused by pain-relief medication are reduction of white blood cells, suppression of the immune system, skin rashes, anemia, dizziness, headache, fatigue, reduction of vision.

The use of pharmaceuticals in arthritis only covers up the symptoms. Just like when it is a rainy day and the roof is leaking, we place a container under the leak to catch the rain for a temporary fix, not thinking to find the hole and patch it. In another example, there is a hole in your wall during the winter, letting in the cold. Not knowing where the hole is, you patch up the entire wall instead of finding the hole and fixing it.

This treatment method (the continual intake of medication) is neither scientifically nor logically acceptable, but it is a fact. We must use the medication because there is no other solution, according to modern medical philosophy.

It is important to note that at one point in time, Western medicine was not in the mainstream because it lacked effectiveness. People had to rely on traditional forms of healing, such as taking herbs and practicing general preventive health measures. It was not until the invention of the microscope that physicians discovered the presence of microorganisms, bacteria, and other pathological substances. From that crucial point on, the body of Western medical knowledge expanded as much information was collected pertaining to biology, science, and the human body. It was because Western medicine was able to see what TCM was unable to see that it reigned superior to TCM, and became the dominant form of medicine.

The following is a statement by Jade Huang on the effects of Western medication compared to those of Eastern medicine.

The 82-year-old patient complained of a minor digestive problem—a perfectly normal complaint for one so old in age. Upon being sent to the hospital, the doctor administered a set dosage of barium to the patient. The ingested barium fluoresces under x-rays so that when the doctor examines the patient's x-rays, he or she may find the cause of the ailment.

Regardless of the patient's age, doctors must issue the same amount of barium in order to reach a conclusion.

The effect of barium on this 82-year-old weak, frail woman was a lapse into coma, spouting of blood, and eventually death. I listened in shock and horror as the news of this patient's death arrived by phone. Eventually, I settled into a state of fury as I realized that my grandmother had died at the hands of doctors who were pretending to cure her.

Where modern Western medicine failed to even diagnose my grandmother's condition, traditional Chinese medicine (TCM) might have correctly diagnosed her condition, cured her of the complaint, and prevented an unnecessary death.

It is my belief that a health care system comprised of modern Western medicine and TCM combined would benefit each individual patient, and ultimately, all of public health. To incorporate the best of both modern Western medicine and TCM, we must first examine their differences—their advantages and disadvantages.

Chapter 7

Traditional Chinese Medicine

How is TCM different?

First of all, modern medicine and TCM differ in the way they view the human body. According to Ted J. Kaptchuk, in his book *The Web That Has No Weaver*, modern medicine is based upon a scientific, systematic, and analytic approach to the human body. The Western physician starts with a symptom, then searches for the underlying mechanism—a precise cause for a specific disease."

Doing so often leads to "analyzing pathology at the cellular and molecular levels," says Katsutoshi Terasawa, *[The Role of Traditional Chinese Medicine in Contemporary Health Care in Japan]*. According to Terasawa, this in turn leads to elucidating general pathology. Oftentimes, however, having broken up the body into such small parts in order to understand them so analytically, the organic nature of the body is forgotten and 'reparative health care' is arbitrary.

After what Terasawa calls "uniform and mass treatment," the physician is unable to predict the patient's special reaction to the medication or treatment. This is due to his failure to recognize each patient's individuality. Each patient differs in constitution, e.g., body condition and degree of seriousness. Accordingly, each patient will react differently to the same pathological process. For example, "infection with the same pathogen may not produce an identical clinical picture in two different patients."

In addition, Western physicians administer treatment in order to control, change, or destroy the pathogen. Oftentimes, this requires chemical intervention, which is followed by side effects. Technological innovations also have this problem. Surgical treatment, for example, although lifesaving and necessary for disorders such as intestinal obstruction due to twisting, has negative aspects as well. Some ramifications include physical pain, danger to the patient's life, the possibility of postoperative infection, and complications. So says Hsien-Chung Wu [*Creating a New Chinese Medicine and Pharmacology*].

Traditional Chinese Medicine [TCM] is based on several thousand years of human experience, and a long line of clinical experience. It has accumulated bit by bit. Chinese medical treatment focuses on the whole person, not just the illness. Illness is only one indication of an imbalance that exists in the whole person. TCM is a holistic form of medicine—that is, it treats the whole person, not just his or her physical condition.

The Chinese physician directs his or her attention to the complete physiological and psychological individual. Each illness affects the whole body, since good health represents a condition of equilibrium in the whole organism. Traditional Chinese physicians never seek to identify a virus. Instead, they view the disease as a disharmony of the body, and they attempt to bring the body back into balance.

The TCM approach to diagnosis reflects that the question of cause and effect is always secondary to the overall pattern. One does not ask, "What X is causing Y?" but rather, "What is the relationship between X and Y?" The Chinese are interested in discerning the relationships among bodily events occurring at the same time. The logic of Chinese medicine attempts to organize the symptoms and signs into understandable configurations. The total configurations, the patterns of disharmony, provide the framework for treatment. The therapy then attempts to bring the configuration into balance, to restore harmony to the individual.

TCM recognizes that each person is specific and thus, responds with personalized treatments catered to the specificity of each patient's condition. This is accomplished by approaching the patient from several points of view and by using the four methods of diagnosis, which are:

1. Observation,
2. Auscultation & Olfaction,
3. Interrogation, and
4. Palpation.

In diagnosing, there are certain points you must keep in mind and specific symptoms you need to watch out for. In addition, you must have a fair knowledge of the meridians and *Yin* and *Yang* principles in order to make correct observations and diagnose diseases.

1. Key Points of <u>Observation</u>
The Chinese physician endeavors to see the patient's "spirit" and discern if he is hyper-or hypo-functional; is in the acute or chronic stage of development; is in high spirits or depressed; is hysterical, semiconscious, restless, quiet, talkative, sad, or irritable.

He will note other distinguishing characteristics as well: the patient's overall body construction, i.e. fat, thin, large, small skeleton, deformities, curled posture, sprawled. He will note characteristics of the extremities: numbness, muscular atrophy, joint inflammation, aches, flexion, range of motion.

The Eastern practitioner will also examine the posture of the patient. Is it meek, proud, curled, sprawled? Does the patient exhibit pain or excess energy? He will observe whether the skin color is bright, glowing, dull, or some other coloration. He'll see if the skin condition is dry, wet, itchy, clear, or has pimples, spots or scars. In addition, he'll check the color of eyes, lips, face, tongue, and nails.

2. Auscultation and Olfaction

In Chinese medicine, auscultation and olfaction make up one entity known as *wen*. Auscultation, or diagnosis by listening, includes listening to the sound and pitch of the voice, cough, breathing, vomiting, hiccup, borborygmi [intestinal rumblings caused by the movement of gas], groaning and other sounds emitted by the patient. In general, a loud sound indicates an excess pattern, while a weak sound indicates a deficient pattern.

According to TCM, voice is associated not only with the vocal organs, but also with the function of *qi*, mainly the *zong qi* or pectoral *qi*. Since the lung dominates respiration and the kidney receives *qi* from the lung, the lung and kidney, therefore, are associated with the strength of voice. By listening to voices and sound, the physician can inspect and detect changes in the vocal organs, internal organs, and the state of any pathogen.

In addition to auscultation, the second part of the four-method diagnosis also includes olfaction. Olfaction refers to smelling any abnormal odor the patient may have. Odors may come from the breath, perspiration, sputum, spittle, nasal discharge, stool, urine, menses, leukorrhea, or other sources.

In general, fetid secretion and excretion pertains to excess syndrome, heat syndrome, or damp heat syndrome. For example, foul smell from the mouth indicates stomach fire. Foul, sour-smelling stools or diarrhea with abdominal pain and rapid pulse result from retention of food and indicate damp heat in the lower intestine. A less foul smell of secretion or excretion indicates a deficient type of syndrome due to cold. Excess syndrome type is due to cold damp.

Body odors are associated with the Five Elements, i.e., rancid for Liver, scorching for Heart, fragrant for Spleen, rotten for Lung, and putrid for Kidney. The source of the odor should also be traced to determine the locality of the disease.

Here are the most commonly used olfactory terms:

Sputum-hot: thick, yellow, smelly—like metal or fish
Sputum-cold: white, thin, bubbly, no smell
Perspiration-hot: smells strong
Urine-hyper: thick, yellow, smells
Urine-hypo: thin, white no smell, cold
Feces-hot: black, dark, strong smell
Feces-cold: soft and loose, light brown
Female discharge-hot: thick, clots, cervical discharge,
    pain, numb, sharp cramps
Female discharge-cold: thin, menses a little late, menses
    a little early

3. **Inquiry or Interrogation**
Inquiry is the chief diagnostic method of learning about the patient's condition. Standard questions of examination relate to:

the patient's present symptoms and history of his/her
illness past medical history [i.e., medication, hospital-
ization]
personal life history
family history
bodily reaction to the environment [i.e. temperature
changes] aches, numbness, pains
urinary and bowel conditions
digestion
trunk/ chest/ abdominal pain
sexual irregularities.

Inquiry should be a step-by-step process. In order to avoid inconsistencies between interrogated information and the actual condition of the patient, the physician should not ask leading questions or the patient may be induced to say what the physician desires to hear.

During an inquiry, the physician should speak in simple language instead of using medical terms. The physician is expected to make his inquiry with the utmost concentration and patience. His expressions should be natural and he should not sigh or show surprise.

4. Palpation:

Palpation is a method of diagnosis in which any pathological condition is detected by palpating, feeling and pressing certain areas of the body to learn of local abnormal changes. This method is divided into two categories:

1.   pulse taking, and
2.   touching different parts of the body.

Pulse Taking: The physician will feel the patient's arterial pulse with his fingers. Pulse taking can reveal the condition of the Zang and Fu organs, qi and blood, and is helpful to judge the location and nature of disease. It also exhibits the prosperity or decline of the vital qi and pathogenic factors to deduce the prognosis of the disease, and to provide the basis for treatment.

Some examples of pulse taking and its indications are:

If pulse is rapid: A quick rate with more than five beats per breath [more than 90 beats per minute] indicates Heat syndromes.

Slippery [or rolling pulse]: Feels smooth and flowing like pearls rolling on a dish. It indicates retention of phlegm and fluid, food retention, excess heat and blood stasis in the lower Jiao [lower part of the body, including the large intestine, urinary bladder, and kidney].

Slippery/rapid pulse: Indicates phlegm fire or food retention, damp-heat or excess heat.

Method of Palpation

The position of a patient is determined by the part of the body to be examined. Palpation is classified into *superficial palpation* and *deep palpation*.

> **Superficial palpation**: This method is also called the *touching-feeling* examination method. Usually the physician will put his or her finger or palm softly on the site to be palpated and increase pressure gradually. This method is often used to examine a patient's body surface and joints.

> **Deep palpation**: This is also known *as pressing examination method*, i.e., a method used to press the deep tissue or organs with your fingers, or your palm. When doing so, the physician will use his index finger, middle finger and ring finger to push gradually downward. This method is often applied to examine the abdominal cavity, or the deep part of the soft tissues.

The Components of Palpation
Palpation of the Skin

The purpose of skin palpation is to find out whether it is cold, feverish, moist, dry, or even puffy in order to determine the condition of the *Zheng Qi* [or vital *Qi*] and pathogens in conflict with each other. If the skin feels very hot when you first palpate it, but becomes less hot the longer you touch it, then the heat is only superficial.

If the skin does not feel very hot at first but becomes hotter and hotter during your palpation, then the heat is internal. However, cold skin shows an excessive coldness of *yin*, or a deficiency of *yang*. If the four limbs are cold while the chest and belly are feverish, this shows heat syndrome with pseudo-cold syndrome [or true heat/false cold syndrome] because *yin* is kept external by excessive *yang* in the interior.

By palpating the skin gently, you can discover whether the body fluid is excessive or deficient. Edema can be distinguished from *qi* stagnation by pressing the swollen site. It is edema if the site, pressed forcefully, sinks, and does not come up immediately after the pressure is moved. Conversely, *qi* stagnation is the cause if the pressed site comes up immediately after the hand is lifted.

Palpation of the Head and the Neck

Palpation of the neck mainly reveals the presence of scrofula [tuberculosis of the lymphatic glands in the neck], goiter [enlargement of the thyroid gland], and tumor.

These four methods: Observation, Auscultation & Olfaction, Interrogation, and Palpation are used in Traditional Chinese Medicine to diagnose the body's condition. The beauty of TCM treatment is that it helps the body to gain enough strength to fight pathogens by itself, without surgery, and thus ensures that the disease is completely cleared. On the basis of this concept, TCM can treat pathologic conditions of unknown etiology.

On a similar plane, TCM can treat diseases that have no immediate, chemical cure such as the early stages of HIV. Traditional Chinese physicians recognize HIV as a weakness of one's immune system, and thus a severe disharmony of one's body. Applying traditional Chinese diagnostic and healing methods, physicians strengthen the body's immune system and bring the body back into balance. So, while Western physicians look for a chemical cure for HIV, traditional Chinese physicians merely bring the body to a healthy state so that it can fight pathogens on its own.

By allowing the body to fight diseases on its own, TCM allows a low cost, natural healing process, which treats a problem from the root instead of from the branch. Because it tries to cure the underlying problem, TCM is slow, and thus, recovery is gradual. In many ways, TCM is more humane and effective than modern Western medicine, especially in the fields of

VALC

general maintenance, preventive health care, and the treating of diseases in their early stages. However, modern medicine is superior to TCM in treating superficial and local lesions.

It is my belief that the differences between modern medicine and TCM call for integration of the two. Such a system is partially in practice in China—the results of which have shown that using the best of both forms of medicine to heal a patient is more beneficial than using either alone.

One would logically presume that integrating the best of both modern medicine and TCM would be a sound course of action. However, this is more easily said than done. Many obstacles stand in the way. For example, certain aspects of TCM are hard to put into modern scientific terms, and therefore, hard to understand. TCM is based upon the Yin-Yang theory, Eight Principles [Yin and Yang, external and internal, heat and cold, excess and deficiency]; the Five Elements of nature: fire, earth, metal, water, and wood; and Qi [internal energy], blood, body fluids, and spirit.

The philosophical differences between modern medicine and TCM make acceptance difficult. As a result of not understanding these basic concepts of TCM, some Western physicians even believe TCM's effectiveness arises from hypnotic suggestion.

Behind Chinese medicine is the philosophy that man lives between heaven and earth, and is a miniature universe in himself. Living things are thought to be made of material that is considered to belong to the yin, or female, passive aspect of nature. The life functions of living things, on the other hand, are considered to belong to yang, or the masculine, active aspect.

In order to grasp more about TCM, you must understand the meaning of the Six Pathogenic Factors. Wind, cold, dampness, heat, dryness and fire are part of Mother Nature. They are normal weather conditions. Why can they become harmful? Let me begin by explaining the Yin Yang Theory.

Yin Yang Theory

The theory of *yin-yang* prevails through all of TCM. It serves to explain the organic structure, physiological functions and pathological change of the human body, and also to guide clinical diagnosis and treatment.

From prevention to treatment of diseases, *yin* and *yang* are centered and fundamental, unique and important. *Yin-yang* is correspondent—if there is *yin*, then there must be *yang*; just like if there is day, then there must be night, anterior and posterior, left and right. There is an old Chinese saying, "If there is only *yang*, nothing grows. If there is only *yin*, there is no reproduction."

In the condition of all matter there must be contention or conflict with a contrasting aspect, like right and left, day and night, man and woman, etc. Two corresponding persons or items, similar in form, are not able to exist without the other. In the *Internal Classic*, the fifth chapter of *Plain Questions* says, "*Yin* remains inside to act as a guard for *yang*, and *yang* stays outside to act as a servant for *yin*." When this is applied to the human body, *yin* corresponds to nutrient substances and *yang* to functional activities.

A statement in the chapter *Manifestations of Yin and Yang* of the *Illustrated Supplement to the Classified Classics* states, "Without *yang* there would be no production of *yin*; without *yin* there would be no production of *yang*." Therefore we say that the relationship between *yin* and *yang* is opposing yet complementing. They can then be used to describe the changes and variations in all things or properties. This is the Theory of *Yin-Yang*.

Some examples in Nature:

Yang	Yin
Day	Night
Spring	Fall
Summer	Winter
Upper	Lower

Examples in the human body:

Yang	Yin
Back	Abdomen
Superior	Inferior
Energy	Blood

Yin and yang are dependent on each other and consume each other. For example, if energy is yang, then blood must be yin. The yin [blood] runs inside your meridians and the yang [which is qi or energy] runs outside your meridians. Both have to check on each other and circulate throughout our whole body. If they do, then we are balanced and everything will be just fine. This balance in the body is vital to our health, and explains the Yin Yang Theory. The Inner Classic emphasizes this point in saying: "Qi is the commander of the blood and blood is the mother of the qi."

The Six Pathogenic Factors

Now that we understand a little about yin and yang, let's talk about the six pathogenic factors, which can cause an imbalance in the body, and open the door to illness.

The passage of the seasons and changes in the weather can have an influence on the human body. Traditional Chinese healers believe that harm is caused by outside pathogenic factors invading. These factors are:

Wind

Cold

Dampness

Heat

Dryness

Fire

Among these six pathogenic factors, wind, cold and dampness are the most common causes of joint "sickness," or arthritis.

Why do these conditions invade our joints? Pathogenic factors are originally normal environmental factors. When human immune systems are weak, or according to TCM, "*Zang qi is insufficient*," then pathogens can invade the body and cause illness. *Zang* means *organ*. Each organ has its own *qi*. So when *zang qi is insufficient*, the organs themselves are deficient, causing a weakening of the immune system. Sometimes a single pathogenic factor invades the body, other times it may be accompanied by other factors or a whole group of other factors. Therefore the sicknesses can be varied and complex.

Wind

Sometimes we say that wind is the source of a hundred diseases. The wind likes to move around, and come and go. In TCM we call it *yang* evil or *excess* evil. Many diseases, in the beginning, have the characteristics of wind evil—headache, skin rash, itch, measles, swelling of the arteries. They all come and go and change quickly—this is all proof of the wind invading.

Cold

Cold is *yin* evil. It easily hurts human *yang qi* [positive energy]. It causes *qi* stagnation and blood obstruction. Proof of cold evil invading is seen in pale facial color, blue, dark or purplish skin color, cold skin temperature, numbness, pain, aversion to cold, fever, absence of sweat, cough, stuffy nose, upper and lower back soreness, frequent urination.

Dampness

Dampness is *yin* evil. It is characterized by stickiness, and can be caused by walking in water, rain, living in a damp area, by eating certain types of food or a malfunctioning digestive system—where your digestive system is not able to transform and transport your food properly. Dampness manifests as aversion to cold; fever; head and body heaviness; soreness in the four limbs; tightness in the chest; lack of thirst; thin white tongue coating; dizziness; blurred vision; fullness in the abdomen. All of these are proof that damp evil is invading.

Heat and Fire

Heat and fire are similar. Other than the degree of heat, they are the same. Fire is extremely hot, so when there is extreme heat it becomes fire. Generally speaking we say that heat evil and fire evil belong to *yang* evil. Fire flames upward when it is severe. Just as the fire burns the forest and spreads out quickly, fire evil represents tidal fever. Tidal fever is called that because the patient's fever recurs daily like the regular rise and fall of the tide. Tidal fever, heat, burning, red face, red eyes, thirst, cold preference, constipation, dark red urine, skin rash, swelling, pus, all are proof that heat evil has invaded.

The six external pathogenic factors are not the only causes of illness. Internal factors can also have an effect. If mood changes within the individual are too extreme, they can harm good health. Seven emotions: happiness, anger, worry, pensiveness, grief, fear and surprise can also cause an imbalance in the body.

To summarize, according to TCM, disease can be caused by:
injury
wind
rain
cold
summer heat
dampness

dryness
yin and yang imbalance
angry or happy emotion
excitement
improper food intake
living in an improper area
being scared or frightened

All of these internal and external factors can cause change or block-ages in our body's inner environment. Consequently, the qi and blood are not able to circulate in the whole person to nourish all four limbs and all the joints, and sickness and pain can appear.

Qi and Blood

Qi is fundamental. You can think of it as oxygen, air, energy, or just simply call it qi. It is composed of **Prenatal Qi**, plus the three elements listed below. Prenatal qi is original qi, or what you are born with. What is referred to in TCM as yuan-qi is transmitted by parents to children at conception. It is one's inherited constitution, and it is stored in the kid-neys.

1) **Grain Qi**, which is developed from digestion of food to produce energy. In TCM it is called Gu-Qi.

2) **Natural Qi**. Every day we breathe in and out. The lungs remove carbon dioxide from the blood and exchange it with oxygen. In TCM this energy ex-change is called Kong-Qi.

3) **Wei Qi,** which is also from food, circulates outside the vessels to protect muscular surfaces, defend the body against outside pathogenic factors, control the opening or closing of pores, moisten skin and

hair, adjust body temperature. It is a TCM belief
that *Wei Qi* is the body's first defense system.

Qi is the source of all movement in the body, therefore without entering and exiting there is no development; without ascending and descending there is no transformation, absorption and storing.

The *Inner Classic* says:
> *Qi is the root of the human body.*
> *Qi dominates warming.*
> *The existence of the antipathogenic Qi in the interior pre-*
> *vents the pathogenic factor from invading.*
> *Qi is transformed from Essence.*
> *Qi is the commander of blood.*
> *The bladder stores body fluid. When the fluid is excreted, the*
> *bladder needs the activities of Qi to help.*

Blood

There are three syndromes relating to blood:
1. Deficiency of blood
2. Heat in the blood, and
3. Stagnation of blood.

Blood is a red liquid that circulates through the vessels and nourishes
the body. It circulates inside meridians and stays inside the vessels to maintain and nourish the system. Blood originates from food essence produced
by the spleen / stomach. It requires the heart to pump it throughout the
body, and the liver to store it. If one of these components were missing,
there would not be single drop of blood produced.

The *Inner Classic* says:
> *When the middle jiao receives food essence it will transform*
> *it into red fluid, which is called blood.*
> *Ying-Qi flows into the vessels to be transformed into blood.*

If blood is not consumed, it turns into essence stores in the
kidney; if essence does not leak out, it is transformed
into blood stored in the liver.

Blood dominates nourishment and moisture.

When the liver receives blood, it gives rise to vision; when the
feet receive blood they are capable of walking; when the
palms receive blood they are capable of holding; and
when the fingers receive blood they are capable of grasping.

When the blood is in harmony . . . the tendons and bones
will be strong and the joints will function smoothly.

Qi and blood are the foundation for human mental activities.

Harmonious circulation of blood ensures a vigorous spirit.

These two fundamentals, *qi* and blood, must be able to circulate
freely for the body to remain harmonized and healthy. You may notice the
following symptoms, which relate to conditions of imbalance:

Deficiency of Qi:

Symptoms: Dizziness, blurring of vision, dislike of speaking, lassitude, spontaneous sweating.

Causes: Long duration of weakness or illness, lacking proper diet, old age,
excess of strain or stress.

Stagnation of Qi:

Symptoms: Distension and pain.
Causes: Mental depression, improper diet, invasion of outside pathogenic
factors, or sprains and strains of muscle.

Deficiency of blood:
<u>Symptoms</u>: Pallor or sallow complexion, pale lips, dizziness, blurring of vision, palpitations, insomnia, numbness of the hands and feet.
<u>Causes</u>: Weakness of spleen / stomach, insufficient material to finish efforts of digestion.

Stagnation of blood:
<u>General symptoms</u>: Weakened or disappearing pulse beat, heaviness, soreness or weakness of the affected limb, difficulty walking, lassitude, fullness of the chest, poor appetite, pale, purplish tongue with a thin coating, dizziness, tiredness, thirsty but don't want to drink, restlessness, headache, palpitations, moodiness, feeling emotional, insomnia. Other symptoms can be pain, mass tumors, hemorrhage, and discoloration of the skin, as in bruising, or spots on the skin.

<u>Causes</u>: Sprains and contusions; hemorrhage; retardation of *Qi* circulation leading to retardation of blood circulation; deficiency of *Qi*, causing a weakness in the normal movement of blood; invasion of pathogenic cold or heat; chronic sickness; congenital weakness; chronic blood loss; overwork, inadequate exercise, overeating of pungent and flavored food.

No matter whether blood stagnation is caused by direct or indirect factors, it will lead to blockage of the blood vessels and absence of pulse beat. Here we are talking about the most common type of blood stagnation: cold, dampness, sprain and weakness in the kidney. The combination will result in lower backache.

Case study:
A 50-year-old woman complained of acute sprain of her lower back. This was not the first time, as she had had attacks three years prior. The first attack occurred after lifting a heavy desk. The present attack happened when she had go to the bathroom, tried to turn, and experienced a severe pain on the right side around the sacroiliac area. The pain radiated down to buttock and leg.

The woman's tongue was slightly red with a greasy coating, with a crack line down the center. Her pulse was wiry and rapid.

Diagnosis: Deficiency of the kidney for a long time, plus cold and damp invasion of the body, causing stagnation of blood. Mixed conditions are the result: dull mass pain, blood stagnation at lower back, causing it to ache.

The following are some of the acupuncture points, herbs and general method I used to assist her.

Treatment and principle:
Eliminate phlegm, resolve dampness, stop the pain and circulate the collaterals.

Acupuncture points:
GB34. Yang Ling Quan [reducing method]
ST36. ZuSan Li [reinforcing method]
ST 41. Jie Xi [even method]
GB30. Huan Tiao [reducing method]

Points at the back:
Extra Hua Tuo Jia Ji [even method]
BL 23. Shen Shu [reinforcing method]
BL 20. Pi Shu [reinforcing method]
Bl 54. Zhi Bian [even method]

Class of Medicinal Herbs:
Here are some herbs I used:
Zhi Ke [Fructus aurantii]
Ban xia [Rhizoma pinelliae]
Chen Pi [Pericarpium citri reticulatae]
Di Long [Lumbricus]
YiYi Ren [Semen coicis]

Du Zhong [Cortex eucommiae]
Dang Gui [Radix angelicae sinensis]
Huang Bai [Cortex phellodendri]
Huang Qi [Radix astragali membranacei]
Bu Gu Zhi [Fructus psoraleae]

How does this all relate to arthritis? Arthritis can manifest as acute or chronic pains, soreness, tiredness, muscles swelling. Tissues, joints and structure are all related in the clinical point of view. Arthritis is inflammation in the body—explained in TCM as being due to wind, cold, dampness invading. But different names or titles are given to differing characteristic signs or locations to differentiate them from others, such as *bursae, synoviae, capsulae, sheets, degenerative, metabolic, neuralgia, neuritis, polyneuritis, syringomyelia, multiple sclerosis, muscular dystrophy, nyasthenia, and peripheral vascular diseases, etc.*

Deficiency of blood and *qi*, or stagnation of *qi* and blood, open the door to an attack by wind, cold, dampness, or a combination of these factors. If, moreover, the invasion cannot be stopped, and infection, genetic deficiency, abnormal or harmful environmental factors or stress are added to the mix, all will gradually develop to affect a deeper level. According to TCM belief, the five external tissues of Vascular, Tendon, Muscle, Skin, and Bone are related to the five internal organs of Heart, Liver, Spleen, Lung, and Kidney.

Treatment & principles:
To promote circulation of *qi*/blood through the meridians and to relieve the pain or disorder, acupuncture and moxibustion are effective. To treat deficiency of blood and *qi*, or nourish the liver and kidney, we apply the Five Element Theory [more explanation later in this chapter]. According to the Five Element theory, the kidneys belong to the so-called water organs, supplying the foundation or basis of a body fluid. The liver is a wood organ—trees are chopped to make fire. After wood is burned, it becomes dust, or earth. Then the good quality substance surface of the

earth is ready for development and growth again. That's the basis of the Five Element theory.

Now, we understand that *qi* and blood both are functional activities of the body. *Qi is the commander of blood, and blood is the mother of qi.* *Qi* and blood are the foundation for human mental activities, and cannot be separated from each other. Therefore, deficiency of *qi* leads to deficiency of blood; or deficiency blood leads to deficiency of *qi*. For this reason when treating disorders related to blood deficiency, *qi* tonics are added to the prescription, or the other way around. If *qi* and blood both are deficient, then restoring both and increasing body tone are absolutely essential.

Acupuncture points in general to restore *qi* and blood:
Basic points:
TW5 . Wei Guan, BL 12. Feng Men.
Sp9. Yin Ling Quan. GB34. Yang Ling Quan.
SP10. Xue Hai.
Upper limbs:
LI15. Jian Yu. TW14. Jian Liao.
LI11. Qu Qi.
Lower limbs:
GB30.Huan Tiao. GB39. Xuan Zhong.
ST35. Du Bi
Back points:
Extra. Hua Tuo Jia Ji [17x2] area.
BL 40. Wei Zhong. BL 60. Kun Lun

Class of Medicinal Herbs:
For stagnation of Qi and blood in general:
Qiang Huo. [Radix et rhizoma notopterygii]
Du Huo. [Radix angelicae pubescentis]
Qin Jiao. [Radix gentianae macrophyllae]
Sang Zhi. [Ramulus mori]
Hai Feng Teng. [Caulis piperis]

Dang Gui. [Radix angelicae sinensis]
Chuan Xiong. [Rhizoma ligustici chuanxiong]
Ru Xiang. [Resina olibani]
Mu Xiang. [Radix Aucklandiae]
Rou Gui. [Cortex cinnamomi]
Mi Zhi Gan Cao. [Radix glycyrrhizae cum melle tosta]

For deficiency of blood and qi or to nourish the liver and kidney:
Formula: "Shi Quan Da Bu Tang Jia Jian"
Ren Shen. [Radix ginseng]
Zhi Huang Qi. [Radix astragali membranacei melle tosta]
Shu Di Huang. [Radix rehmanniae praeparata]
Dang Gui. [Radix angelicae sinensis]
Gui Zhi. [Ramulus cinnamomi]
Dan Shen. [Radix salviae miltiorrhizae.]
Fu Ling. [Sclerotium poriae albae]
Ji Xue Teng. [Caulis et radix millettiae seu spatholobi]
Mi Zhi Gan Cao. [Radix glycyrrhizae melle tosta]

Five Elements Theory

The Five Elements Theory is the backbone of TCM philosophy.
It symbolizes how the internal organs associate and communicate with others, and how they work as a group.

The theory of the five elements corresponds in nature to wood, fire, earth, metal and water equivalent as liver, heart, spleen, lung, and kidney. These elements are in a state of constant motion and change. This theory was first formed in China around 221 BC. It derives from observations of the natural world made in early times by the Chinese people in the course of their lives and productive hard work.

Five elements: Kidney [water], liver [wood], heart [fire], spleen/stomach [earth], lung [metal], were considered to be five essential materials for the maintenance of life and production. The water nourishes the tree, the tree grows, and provides timber for burning, for fuel, for energy, or other material. The heart is a fire organ, like a chamber or enclosed compartment for heating, baking, for firing, baking, hardening, when something is burned. The grayish-white to black powdery residue left after burning becomes earth or soil [spleen/stomach]. We mine metal [lung] from deposits of ore or minerals in the earth. When we set the metal in a corner, it will become moist from air condensing onto cool metal surfaces and that produces water [kidneys]. So water nourishes the wood, the wood becomes a log, heart sets up the fire, the burning leaves ash, ash becomes land, inside the land is mining, and that creates water.

The circle contributes to the progress or growth—able to extend life. In TCM we call it a *generation cycle*, or *promotion cycle*.

In this theory, food relies on water and fire; production relies on metal and wood; earth gives birth to everything. People used all these elements in their daily lives.

In TCM, this theory is generally and universally applicable. It explains the nature of the *zang-fu* organs and the inter-relationships between them, and the relation between human beings and the natural world to guide clinical diagnosis and treatment. That's the basis of the Five Elements Principle and methods.

An example of the Five Elements Theory in operation relates to growth. Growth means to allow something to develop or reproduce, to spread, to gradually intensify, to become smaller or to make something pleasurable and acceptable. These are all completely fundamental phenomena—the natural or real aspect of a person, place, or thing.

Harmony refers to a complementary relationship such as mutual understanding, or *yin and yang* balance. The Five Elements Theory explains the natural behavior or specific set of phenomena that relates to everything. After the earth provides us with food, we need metal, maybe an axe, for felling trees or chopping wood, in order to make fire. After wood is burned, it becomes ash or dust, or Earth. Later it becomes a solid surface.

The earth supplies the floor of a body of water, and the circle begins again. All these elements must be in harmony to complete the cycle. Those are the basics of the Five Elements Theory I'm talking about.

All of the many elements of the human body must be working in harmony for complete health. Most people don't understand anything about the inner working of their bodies. This lack of knowledge often causes them to take advice from health practitioners that may not be in their best interests. Their total body function is not taken into consideration. People are fearful when problems occur, and this fear can add overload to an already debilitated system. It is very important to overcome this reaction. If you research your subject, you know your enemy—you become unafraid of it. Then you can take the path toward your recovery that best suits your situation.

Did you know that even your body's water metabolism will influence internal and external elements such as whether you are happy, angry, worried, sad, afraid, grieving? Water metabolism also affects wind, cold, rain, summer heat, and dampness influence. In addition to your water balance, many, many other factors can have an effect on your body's equilibrium: chemical imbalances, lack of certain nutrients, toxicity from an improper diet, lack of sleep, too much stress, and on and on.

It is just like the *Inner Classic* says, "Hundred diseases are beginning, wind, rain, cold, summer. *Yin and yang*, happy and angry, diet, living space, big shock or sudden fright causes *qi* and blood to separate. *Yin and yang's* relationship is broken, and the meridians become blocked."

Chapter 8

What is Acupuncture?

It's simple. Any number of factors can influence your body's balance, which blocks your meridians, and when this happens, disease can occur. Once your body has fallen into a diseased or unharmonious state, what can you do to help it recover? One solution is to try acupuncture.

What is Acupuncture?

One of the main components of TCM, acupuncture as been a conventional therapy in China for close to 3,000 years. It is believed that all your internal structures, systems and organs are connected to *meridians* or channels. If one of more of these 14 channels are out of balance or blocked, your body may react in different ways—sometimes with illness or pain.

How does sticking a needle in your body help you? According to TCM principles, this needle, inserted into certain points along the meridians, can stimulate your body to open the pathways of *qi* (life energy) that flow through your body, and adjust the imbalances. Acupuncture concentrates the body's self-healing powers in the points where it is needed.

Let's say that your cells, size-wise, are like ants (actually they are much, much, much smaller than ants). To these ants, an acupuncture needle looks just like a big giant tree. When the acupuncture needle is inserted in your body, it's like a tree is stuck right in the middle of the highway. Because a foreign object has penetrated your body, your white cells, your soldiers, have to respond. Your central command center (central nervous system) sends a message to the soldiers, saying go ahead—carry all your artillery, all your heavy equipment, and get rid of the enemy.

These needles come into our body, and our soldiers (white cells or T-cells) don't know anything about acupuncture. Our physical body, micro-organisms, cells—none of these know what these acupuncture needles are—they just know that a foreign body has penetrated, and must be fought. So the needles penetrate in different places, and they get different responses.

Our body has to accumulate certain power and make sure we have supplies, transportation, and ammunition. Acupuncture provokes not only a local reaction, but everywhere else in the body too. While the soldiers are rushing to defend their posts, they make your body alert. They carry the power from place A to place B to reach the needle's location, and on the way, they have to fix the problems they encounter. They have to clear the debris from the road, otherwise their trucks cannot go through. Maybe the needle is in the east, and the soldiers are living in the west—a long way to travel. While they travel they fix the highway, make the communication good, etc.

Consequently, our body gets the benefit. While all the artillery and heavy equipment is on the way, the soldiers have to repair the roads, build the bridges, feed the troops—everything to enable the army to fight the enemy. That's why acupuncture works.

What To Expect From Acupuncture Treatment

What exactly will acupuncture do in my body?

Harmonize *yin and yang*, according to the *yin/yang* theory.

Regulate the meridians (meridian theory): 12 muscular regions, 15 collaterals, 12 divergent meridians, 12 cutaneous regions, root and branch origins and ends.

De Qi sensation is the key of success. *Qi* must arrive in the local area as well as around the area of illness. The patient should feel soreness, numbness, swelling and heaviness.

Technical and clinical skills are important: needles are the acupuncturist's extension of his mind and arms. Diagnosis is primarily applied from an understanding of a disease's signs and symptoms.

The Procedure

Your TCM practitioner or acupuncturist will determine how many needles should be inserted in your body, and at what points. This always depends upon your specific situation. The needles are very, very thin, and are usually placed in the area of pain at points in the arms and legs. The TCM view of disease is that there is an imbalance or blockage of *qi* (life force). The painful area represents the blockage of *qi*, and points in the extremities are used to balance the *qi*.

Needle insertion feels somewhat like a mosquito bite, depending on your sensitivity to pain. The most sensitive areas are on the skin surface; once the needle penetrates the skin there is usually no more pain.

Only disposable needles are used to avoid transmission of AIDS or other infectious diseases.

Once the needles are in place you must lie still for 10-15 minutes. Movement with needles may cause discomfort, so make sure you are very comfortable before the treatment begins. This is also time for you to let go of any pain you may be unconsciously holding onto.

After the treatment you may feel very relaxed because of the release of endorphins (the body's natural morphine-like painkillers).

Another philosophy has two basic ways of looking at diseases: they may be *mechanical* or *energetic*. A *mechanical* disease means there is some difficulty moving the body: neck pain, back pain, arm or leg pain, etc. There are many causes such as over-use of certain muscles, trauma (injury from an accident), degeneration from over-use or aging. *Energetic* disease means there is some internal organ system imbalance causing these disease processes. Many times what appears to be simply mechanical may be of internal origin. The acupuncture system is designed to treat both—the mechanical (external appearance of symptoms) and the energetic (internal cause).

The best results are accomplished in a series of 5-10 treatments, usually administered once or twice each week depending on the severity of the problem. Full balancing of your body's internal or energetic properties may take longer and require additional herbal supplements.

Acupressure, needles, laser, electric stimulation, *moxibustion* (heat therapy) and cupping are also extensions of the acupuncturist's mind and body. Herbal combinations, in the form of tablets or tea, are also tools which an acupuncturist can use to assist a patient.

It may be necessary to change your diet or lifestyle in order to get the best outcome. The ancient ways may not show instant results, but it has been my experience that a gradual improvement is likely, and can ultimately reverse or relieve your symptoms in a more natural manner than drugs or surgery.

General acupuncture treatments for common syndromes

Common Treatment Methods: Depending on which factor is predominant, we must choose the proper therapeutic method to treat it, such as expel wind, dispel damp, disperse cold, clear the heat, nourish dryness, purge fire.

Expel wind. Wind is the primary exogenous pathogenic factor in causing diseases. It is a *yang* pathogenic factor and is characterized by "upward and outward dispersion." Wind in nature blows in gusts and is characterized by rapid changes. Wind is characterized by constant movement.

Acupuncture points to expel wind:
LI 4. He Gu. TW5. Wai Guan.
GB20. Feng Qi. BL12. Feng Men.
GB31. Feng Shi.

Method: reducing method. Moxibustion may be used to warm and circulate the channels.

Class of Medicinal Herbs to expel wind:
Ge Gen [Radix puerariae]
Zhi Ma Huang [Herba ephedrae melle tosta]
Gui Zhi [Ramulus cinnamoni]
Fang Feng [Radix ledbouriellae]
Sang Zhi [Ramulus mori]
Wei Ling Xian [Radix clematidis]

Qin Jiao [Radix gentianae macrophyllae]
Qi Shao Yao [Radix paeoniae rubrae]
Bei Xie [Rhizoma dioscoreae hypoglaucae]
Cang Zhu [Rhizoma atractylodis]
Han Fang ji [Radix stephaniae tetrandrae]

Dispel damp. Damp is characterized by heaviness and turbidity, viscosity and stagnation. It is a *yin* pathogenic factor that impairs *yang* and easily obstructs *Qi* circulation.

Acupuncture points to Dispel Damp:
TW 6. Zhi Gou LI10. Shou San Li.
ST40. Feng Long. GB34. Yang Ling Quan.
ST36. Zu San Li SP9. Yin Ling Quan.
SP6. San Yin Jiao.

Method: reducing method. Moxibustion may be added if cold symptoms are predominant.

Class of Medicinal Herbs to dispel damp:
Mu Gua. [Fructus chaenomelis]
Yi Yi Ren. [Simen coicis]
Wu Jia Pi [Cortex acanthopanacis radicis]
Shen Jin Cao [Herba lycopodii clavati]
Lu Lu tong [Fructus liquidambaris]
Tu Fu Ling [Rhizdoma smilacis glabrae]
Sang Zhi [Ramulus mori]
Si Gua Luo [Fasciculus vascularis luffae]
Qin Jiao [Radix gentianae macrophyllae]
Qiang Huo [Rhizoma et radix notopterygii]
Du Huo [Radix angelicae pubescentis]
Hai Feng Teng [Caulis pipeeris futokadsureae]
Luo Shi Teng [Caulis trachelospermi]
Wsei Ling Xian [Radix clematidis]

Disperse cold. Cold is a yin pathogenic factor that consumes the yang qi of the body. Cold is characterized by contraction and stagnation, resulting in impairment of the opening and closing of the pores, spasmodic contraction of tendons and channels, and impaired circulation of qi and blood.

Acupuncture points to disperse cold:

TW5. Wai Guan. TW4. Yang Qi.
ST36. Zu San Li. Liv3. Tai Chong.
GB31. Feng Shi. GB34. Yang Ling Quan.

Method: even method, reinforcing method on St 36 (Zu San Li) Moxibustion or heat lamp can be used.

Class of Medicinal Herbs to disperse cold:

Zhi Chuan Wu [Radix aconiti kusnezoffii]
Zhi Cao Wu [Radix aconiti kusnezoffii praeparata]
Zhi Ma Huang [Herba ephedrae melle tosta]
Gui Zhi [Ramulus cinnamoni]
Xi Xin [Herba asari cum radice]
Zhi Fu Zi [Radix aconiti lateralis praeparata]
Rou Gui [Cortex cinnamoni]
Lu Jiao Jiao [Colla cornus cervi]
Chuan Xiong [Rhizoma ligustici chuanxion]
Yin Yang Huo [Herba epimedii]
Ji Xue Teng [Caulis et radix millettiae seu spatholobi]
Dang Gui [Radix angelicae sinensis]
Jiang Huang [Rhizoma curcumae longae]
Du Huo [Radix angelicae pubescentis]

Clear heat / fire [including mild heat and heat]. Heat / fire is a yang pathogenic factor characterized by burning and upward direction. Pathogenic fire often consumes yin fluid. Invasion by fire stirs up interior liver wind and causes disturbance of blood such as nosebleed, blood in the urine, spitting of blood, bloody stool, uterine bleeding, excessive menstrual bleeding, carbuncle, boil and ulcer.

Acupuncture points to clear heat / fire:
LI4. He Gu. LI11. Qu Qi.
GB20. Feng Qi. TW5. Wai Guan.
ST44. Nei Ting. Liv2. Xing Jian.
BL17. Ge Shu.

Method: reducing method. Moxibustion is contraindicated.

Class of Medicinal Herbs to clear heat / fire:
Tu Fu Ling [Rhizoma smilacis glabrae]
Shui Niu Jiao [Cornu bubali]
Sheng Di Huang [Radix rehmanniae recens]
Qi Shao Yao [Radix paeoniae rubrae]
Mu Dan Pi [Cortex moutan radicis]
Ren Dong Teng [Caulis seu ramus lonicerae]
Huang Bai [Cortex phellodendri]
Zhi Mu [Rhizoma anemarrhenae]
Jin Yin Hua [Flos lonicerae]
Lian Qiao [Fructus forsythiae]
Pu Gong Ying [Herba taraxaci cum radice]
Zi Hua Di Ding [Herba violae cum radice]
Di Gu Pi [Cortex lycii radicis]

Nourish dryness: Dryness consumes body fluids, resulting in dryness of the nose and throat, dry mouth with thirst, chapped skin, withered body hair, constipation and reduced urination. Invasion by pathogenic dryness often impairs the function of the Lung, the "delicate" organ, which, like the *Inner Classic* description, has the function of dispersing, descending & moistening.

Acupuncture points to nourish dryness:
CV6. Qi Hai CV4. Guan Yuan.
ST36. Zu San Li. Liv3. Tai Chong.
UB18. Gan Shu. GB34. Yang Ling Quan.
LI4. He Gu.

Method: reinforcing method of CV6. Qi Hai, CV4. Guan Yuan. ST36. Zu San Li; even method on the other points. Moxibustion is applicable, except in case of Heat signs; in some clinical cases deficient patient may have mild heat.

Class of Medicinal Herbs to nourish dryness:
Dang Shen [Radix codonopsis pilosulae]
Huang Qi [Radix astragali membranacei]
Gui Zhi [Ramulus cinnamoni]
Dang Gui [Radix angelicae sinensis]
Chuan Xiong [Rhizoma ligustici chuanxion]
Ji Xue Teng [Caulis et radix millettiae seu spatholobi]
Wu Wei Zi [Fructus schizandrae sinensis]
Hong Hua [Flos carthami]

Purge fire: Fire is characterized by extreme heat, consumption of body fluid or *yin* factor. Drives off or scatters the energy.

Acupuncture points to purge fire:
LI4. He Gu. GB20. Feng Qi.
GV14. Da Zhui. GV20. Bai Hui.
UB12. Feng Men. LI11. Qu Qi.
LU11. Shao Shang. SP10. Xue Hai.
PC5. Jian Shi. LI1. Shang Yang.

Method: reducing method. No moxabustion.

Class of Medicinal Herbs to purge fire:
Da Huang [Rhubarb]
Huang Qin [Scutellaria]
Huang Lian [Coptis]
Huang Bo [Phellodendron]
Shi Gao [Gypsum]
Zhi Zi [Gardenia]

Chapter 9

Prevention of Arthritis

How to Prevent the Onset of Arthritis

Now that we've talked generally about some of TCM's philosophies, let's get back to our subject. How can we prevent arthritis from getting a foothold in the body?

Avoiding arthritis is almost impossible because, like any machine that is used, the body will eventually wear out. However, good maintenance will extend the life of the instrument.

Prediction is a method of prevention

Humans are emotional animals. Very often we realize this, but still we are unable to avoid allowing our emotions to control us. When we allow our emotions to dominate our lives, we find our health is continually being compromised as our moods swing this way and that. If we try to stabilize our emotions, and stop overreacting to every occurrence, our internal health improves immeasurably.

Every person has stress of one kind or another. The key to balance is to avoid allowing the stress to affect you. Each person has to find his or her own way to handle or release these everyday forces.

Prediction is a method of prevention. We cannot always predict how things will work—if this was the case, everything would happen at the same time for every person. What I mean is you have to have some knowledge or expectation of what will happen in a certain circumstance. You predict what will happen next. For example, if you know the weather the next couple of days will be cold or damp or rainy, then you may understand that your joints might have a bad time. How to prevent this? Keep warm, stay indoors—that's what I mean.

We have to be very distinct about what our symptoms or complaints are. For each of the different kinds of arthritis, the causes can be different. If arthritis is beginning to develop in our body, we must be clear about what exactly is happening. In the case of every single disease, we must characterize it, and combine both western and eastern medicine to help us. Or sometimes we have to choose which solution is the best or proper at the time. We must very carefully and sincerely consider each alternative.

The following ideas are a general method of prevention, and a reference for you to consider in your quest to be arthritis-free.

Have a daily exercise routine. Every day you must do some kind of continuous exercise that makes you sweat—for at least 20 minutes. I recommend walking up and down stairs. From my clinical experience, I have found this helps to move all the joints, keeps the body balanced and flexible and also promotes blood circulation. In addition, exercise is extremely important for bone and muscle strength. When muscles are not used, they lose their tone. Strong muscles are important in providing support to joints, and can be built with exercise.

The three types of exercise that are best for people with arthritis are *range of motion* exercises:

1) **Strengthening exercises.** These exercises involve and improve muscular contraction against resistance in which the length of the muscle remains the same. Yoga is a desirable practice for strengthening and promoting control of the body and mind.

2) *Qi Gong* **practice.** *Qi Gong* exercises involve and improve oxygen consumption by the body, promoting energy and blood circulation.

3) **Sweating exercises.** Sweating exercises involve and improve pushing, pulling against resistance, and stretching to build strength and flexibility until sweating out. All these exercises are good, especially for osteoarthritis,

All exercise is beneficial for the joints, weight control, reduction of blood pressure, and generally enhancing wellbeing. Swimming or exercising in water is very good for people with arthritis or inflammation in some joints. Remember to work with qualified physical therapists or certified instructors, to avoid damaging your body.

Keep a proper bodyweight. An overweight body increases your heart overload, and also creates heart and blood vessel problems. At the same time, it is difficult to make your joints accept tremendous unexpected pressure. If you are not careful, you can easily sprain a joint, or traumatize it. Make sure your weight is not more than 20% higher than the accepted standard body weight generally agreed on by most medical professionals.

The biggest reasons for excess weight are lack of exercise and overeating—taking in more calories than needed. Of course sometimes weight can be related to one's heritage, endocrine system, and emotions. They are all closely connected. A person who has no control over his weight should seek professional help.

Be joyful and happy mentally. Nerve, muscle and joint pain and the central nervous system are closely related. In the clinic we see many diseases that we cannot find any causes for, such as mental diseases and mental trauma. These are affiliated with the central control system. Emotional behavior, unsettled feelings, nervousness, weakness in the tendons, excess sweating, and skin eruptions are all signs of a central nervous system problem.

Stabilize your emotions. Avoid anything that can cause tension. Improve and train your central nervous system to protect yourself from neuro-area disease. I recommend meditation, religious activities, soaking baths, singing, dancing, praying, travel, acupuncture or massage. All of these will help relax you mentally.

The rules for prevention of all diseases are:
Drink enough water. Drinking at least eight glasses of water daily will help flush toxins from your cells, hydrate your organs, and maintain a proper balance of your body systems.

Have a daily bowel movement. Everyone needs to have a routine bowel movement every day. If one day something unusual happens, it means that the inside of your body is undergoing some sort of change. We must find out the reason for change.

Generally speaking, the stool should not be too dry or too wet. It should be bigger than your thumb. The length should be longer than your fist, and the best color would be light yellow. Otherwise, you should find out the reasons why it differs from the information here.

A healthy person usually has one daily bowel movement that is easy and pleasant. If there are any diseases influencing the digestion or if there are any digestion problems, the stool will come with a sticky liquid and sometimes some undigested food as well. These are important indications that are very easy to diagnose and understand how our own system is currently functioning.

Good urination. The urine is an important health indicator. From the frequency, volume and the feeling of your urination, you are also able to understand whether or not your body's evaporation functions are normal.

Urination also indicates one's water accumulation condition. Frequent urination and scarce urination are both abnormal. A day's urine output should be more than 400 ml. The sensation of constantly needing to urinate, coming with an urgent feeling of pressure, means there is too much urine.

Either way, when bladder evaporation function is abnormal, it is because the kidneys are unable to *seal* their kidney *qi*. This happens when the person's *low burner* is too cold and is too damp. If the dampness turns to damp heat they always have the sensation of pressure on the bladder. What's the *low burner*? I'll explain later on in this chapter.

What do I mean when I say the kidneys are not able to seal? The kidney is supposed to keep its treasure inside—the sperm, the blood purifiers. These elements should not be allowed to leak out. You need to keep that stuff in a safe area. And seal means lock it in. If the kidney is unable to lock, not able to seal, it allows this treasure to leak out or explode. Your body is broken.

Just like if you put your money in a safe, and there is a hole in the back, all your money falls out. It's easy to steal your money from behind your safety box—it's not sealed properly.

Anyway, back to the need to monitor your urination function. All of the following urination symptoms need to be checked on as soon as possible because they indicate an abnormal condition:

    painful urination
    fullness and being able to urinate
    unable to control urination
    dripping urine
    not being able to urinate

If the patient has too little urine (dark yellow in color) and high body heat, thirst and puffiness, it almost certainly must be edema. This requires urgent medical treatment to prevent the sickness from becoming more severe.

All of the urination symptoms mentioned above are a warning to seek treatment—never underestimate them. The volume of urine, too much or too little, is an important indicating element. If the patient feels thirsty, has a sore knee and mid-section, has cold pains (if he feels like he is sitting down in water from the waist down), and has profuse urine (clear and long) he may be suffering from a wasting disease or he quite probably has diabetes.

Avoid delaying treatment for these symptoms. Don't miss the treatable period.

Good appetite

Good appetite means you enjoy eating all kinds of food—you enjoy everything. You like to eat it. Everything is very tasty. There's no good food, there's no bad food. Appetite relates to how each person consumes food, how you digest it, and how you feel. Good appetite has nothing to do with being hungry—if you are hungry all the time, it could mean that you have a parasite residing inside your colon.

As long as your body is able to consume and to digest, your absorption function is healthy. However, food that is good for you may not be good for me. My body may not be able to digest the same food that you enjoy. Your treasure might be my enemy.

Good digestion and absorption

Food intake and digestion absorption functions are mainly related with the organs of spleen and stomach, liver and gall bladder, large and small intestine, *triple warmer* (see explanation of *triple warmer* later in the chapter). If our food intake cannot be transformed into purified essence, qi and blood to nourish our needs, then the body's physical activity will stop and the human being will lose vitality.

The human body has six *zang* and six *fu* organs, or nighttime and daytime organs. They all have a different mission. The zang organs are mainly working at night; fu organs work during the day. To understand the human body's zang/fu function and activity is very important.

Zang Organs are:
Lung
Spleen
Heart
Kidney
Pericardium
Liver

Fu Organs are:
Large intestine
Stomach
Small intestine
Urinary bladder
Triple warmer (see explanation later in the chapter)
Gall bladder

After a person is born, his stomach dominates the acceptance of nourishment, and the spleen dominates its transformation. These organs create qi and blood, sustaining the zang/fu organs. A TCM belief is that the stomach digests the food, and then gives it to the spleen. The spleen is like the deliveryman—he is supposed to deliver all this food that the stomach has processed to all the departments, to nourish and then in turn create energy and blood.

We know that strong or weak spleen and stomach function mirror the strength or weakness of the body's condition. Therefore we know that we need to guard the spleen and stomach in order to remain strong—using wei qi, as we say in Chinese. Wei qi is protection energy. There is an old Chinese saying, "The four seasons, a hundred diseases. Wei qi is the source of life. You have wei qi and you are alive. No wei qi and you die."

Wei qi has a full mission in your body:
1. To warm your body,
2. Protect your body,
3. Promote your energy,
4. Seal your energy.

These four functions are vital for the body's survival and freedom from disease.

Good sleep.
Sleeping is an important physical activity for human beings. The inability to have a good night's sleep will cause the human body to lose its *yin and yang* balance, normal life activities will lose their rhythm, and one's health will certainly be influenced.

A normal healthy human being has saturated *qi* and blood. *Saturated* means full, just like the full moon, or when the ocean water reaches its highest level. It also means *satisfaction* to the TCM practitioner. So when we say the *qi* and blood are saturated, it means that they are at their fullest potential—everything is balanced. If *yin and yang* are sealed properly, then the brain should be very healthy, the spirit clear and strength full with energy.

Consequently, when sleeping, the brain should be very calm and quiet. The duration of sleep, the sleeping condition, the presence of dreams, and if a person has insomnia or requires more sleep than normal, are all extremely important elements that we should emphasize and consider.

Avoid wind, cold and damp heat invasion. In your living and working area, try to avoid drafts, dampness, cold, or extreme heat, and you will have tolerance. Also, improper dress, such as wet clothes, must be changed out of right away, to maintain your body's ability to avoid invasion by cold dampness. Keep your bed covers clean and dry. Avoid common cold attack by wind, cold and heat. Allow your body *qi* and blood normal function.

Not only must you avoid external cold, dampness, and heat invasion, but also their internal counterparts. Our human body is a small universe, and has internal wind, cold, dampness, and dryness, just like outside. There are interior forces that create these factors also. So you have to work with the outside atmosphere, plus you also have to remain harmonized and internally peaceful. Otherwise the interior will create wind, cold and dampness and those kinds of things.

Here are a few preventive suggestions you can use to avoid wind cold invading your body: Use acupuncture and Chinese herbs to strengthen your spleen to dispel the damp; avoid greasy, fatty foods and alcohol, avoid smoking. Avoid sexual activity—keep your sperm in your body. Avoid dampness and sticky living spaces

Triple Warmer and the Three Burners

At this point, let me digress a little to explain about the body's three burners that we began to talk about in the preceding pages. It is a TCM belief that we have three burners: Upper, Middle, and Lower Burners.

Your *Low Burner* consists of your lower organs–your kidneys, liver, bladder, and large intestine.
Your *Middle Burner* relates to the stomach and spleen.
Your *Upper Burner* is comprised of your brain, heart, and lungs.

99

Your low burner needs to be able to warm up and cook the food. If the low burner is not functioning, you are not able to process what you eat, and the water or urine is not able to evaporate, is not able to steam, is not able to discharge—because the low burner is not strong enough. Your organ fire is not hot enough. Your power is not strong.

In ancient days the Chinese believed the body had these three burners mentioned above—cooking sites. Actually, they do not exist—it is only imagination. In the old days when a person died, the tradition was to bury the person in the ground. Two to three years later, the body would be dug up again. All the flesh would be gone, the bones were still there, but they would find three places on the body that looked like something burned there. That's why they think the human being has three burners inside the body. To complete the traditional religious ritual, they would then place the bones in some kind of clay bucket with a cover, and remove it to a temple.

The Traditional Chinese physician believes the human body has what's called a Triple Warmer Meridian, but we cannot find that there are corresponding organs. From the TCM point of view, the Triple Warmer Meridian is very important. Take, for example, the case of a person who has the symptoms of diabetes (we call this the wasting and thirsting syndrome). If there is a big thirst, we believe it is an upper burner problem. If there is a big hunger, this means the middle burner doesn't work. Frequent urination or profuse urination is considered a low burner problem. Therefore, a person who has diabetes is always diagnosed as wasting, thirsting, upper, middle or lower burner in excess, or maybe all three of them.

A meridian is like a nerve, a path, or a road. From any point in a meridian, one stimulation point, you can connect to the end of the meridian—the last point. We have a meridian for triple warmer, but we don't have the organs. We have a heart meridian, and we have a heart. We have a stomach meridian, and we have a stomach. We have a large intestine meridian, and we have a large intestine. But the triple warmer meridian—

we don't have any organs that relate to it. The ancient Chinese saw the three burned spots there—that's why we believe we have three organs.

Back to triple warmer and diabetes—why is the diabetic person always very hungry and thirsty? The middle burner corresponds to the stomach and spleen. The TCM belief is that if the middle burner doesn't work the food taken in is not cooked, or processed, and the body is not able to absorb the food. It's not properly processed because the pilot light is out. That's why some people are big eaters, but never gain weight.

When one's lower burner is not functioning, meaning the fire is not hot enough, all this stuff remaining in the place becomes very cold, very damp, and then creates lots of problems. In any situation where there is sluggish movement, or blockage, bacteria can invade, and the body's qi is compromised. The body is unbalanced, and all sorts of conditions can be the result, including arthritis.

Chapter 10

Treating Osteoporosis Arthritis

How Natural Herbs and Acupuncture Can Heal Your Arthritis

Bone is unique for its mineralized matrix; on average by weight, it is 65% mineral, and 35% organic tissue. It forms the skeleton of the body. Bone is a reservoir of calcium, and acts as an anchor for muscles, tendons and ligaments. It harbors many internal viscera including the central nervous system; it assists in the mechanism of respiration; and is a center of blood-forming activity and fat storage.

Bone contains calcium, phosphorous, and a small amount of water. Approximately two-thirds of bone is composed of calcium, which makes it hard and brittle. Phosphorous makes up about one-third of bone's elements, and is what makes it pliant. Bone substance is comprised of marrow, *osteoprogenitor* cells, *osteoblasts* (bone forming cells), and bone absorbing cells or *osteoclasts*.

Compact bone is the outer, impact-resistant, weight-bearing shell of bone. It is surrounded on its outer surface by a layer of fibrous connective tissue, called the *periosteum*. The matrix of compact bone occurs in two patterns: concentric layers with a central canal arranged in columns, and layers between and around *haversian* systems. *Haversian* canals are the channels in bone containing blood vessels and nerves.

You can see that bones are not just decoration to give your body an attractive appearance. They are complex multi-functional structures that form your body's frame and support your organs. Bones are dynamic, and are constantly changing. The *osteoclasts* in our bones continually tear down old bone cells, while the *osteoblasts* build new ones. The bones respond to the demands you make upon them, such as carrying a heavier workload, becoming thicker and stronger.

Calcitonin, secreted by the thyroid and parathyroid glands, regulates the *osteoclast* and obstructs the release of calcium from the bones into the blood. *Calcitonin* lowers the calcium concentration in the blood, and also transforms *osteoclast* into *osteoblast*, causing calcium to be stored in the bone. When a person's hormonal balance is disturbed, such as when a woman reaches menopause, the *calcitonin* secretion is also disturbed. This causes the *osteoblasts* and *osteoclasts* to miscalculate, which in turn causes bone substance to be altered.

The *ossification* process (or hardening of bone) is regulated by growth hormones, or may be said to come from the pituitary gland and the sex hormones. It is deeply relative to osteoporosis arthritis. After menopause, women's bodies change because of hormonal differences. As a matter of fact, a woman loses her bone substance and marrow ten times faster than a man does at this age. Her bones become thin and porous. Not only that, but *calcitonin* levels may be closely related to cardiac rhythm, muscular contraction, nervous system activities, blood clotting, and enzyme levels.

Osteoporosis arthritis is a preventable and treatable disease, if you know how. It is often called a "silent" disease because it can progress for years without symptoms before a fracture occurs.

Osteoporosis has primary and secondary causes. The primary cause is natural bone degeneration. Sometimes this is due to the bone formation and resorption processes speeding up, and when bone resorption is more active than bone absorption, calcium salt from the bone is released into the blood. This can lead to breakdown or fracture of the bone.

Why does the bone degenerate? Let me give you a very brief summary of the hormone concern related to osteoporosis arthritis. The pituitary gland is governed by the thalamus and hypothalamus, and is the so-called seat of the regulating centers of the brain. These regulating centers include the autonomic (spontaneous) centers governing the heart, blood pressure, temperature control, acid-alkali balance, and metabolism.

Several sex hormones rule the production of estrogen in the ovaries. When menopause occurs, these hormones produce less estrogen, creating an imbalance, and ultimately, creating less bone substance. The female body changes and osteoporosis arthritis occurs.

The testosterone hormone of the male has similar effects to the female's estrogen. Men, however, suffer from osteoporosis approximately ten years later than a woman of the same age. The decrease in male testosterone is gradual and takes a longer time.

As I said, the primary cause of osteoporosis is bone degeneration from hormonal causes. Secondary causes of osteoporosis are:

> Lifetime inadequate calcium intake.
> Regular intake of high protein foods.
> Over-use of caffeine, soft drinks, or chocolate.
> Insufficient intake of milk, glucose, galactose, whey products.
> Long-time intake of certain medications, such as complex organic acid, used in the treatment of thrombosis to prevent blood clots, antacids, etc.
> Over-use of alcohol and/or cigarettes.
> Persons who have experienced space flight, or other anti-gravity activity.

Stroke, coma, or being in a fixed position and not able to move. This includes lack of exercise, joint injury, fractured limb, immobilized in a cast—anything that impedes limb or body movement.

Osteoporosis is a natural disease—as we age we all acquire it. Nowadays there are many advancements in western medication, however, I feel that ancient Chinese treatment methods are safer and, although sometimes slow, reliable.

General symptoms of Osteoporosis Arthritis

emaciation

hot flush

feeling of warmth

night sweats

heat in the palms and soles

dizziness

tiredness

thirst

restlessness

headache

palpitation

moodiness

emotional feelings

insomnia

numbness of skin

feeling of ants crawling in the body

decrease in body height

Spinal deformity resulting in *kyphosis* (hump) usually at the lumbar and cervical area. Kyphosis causes the patient to bend forward when walking.

Key Symptoms of Osteoporosis Arthritis
    lumbago soreness
    softness of the lower back
    weakness of the knees
    difficulty walking
    weakness of the legs
    lack of force when walking
    pressure and pain felt in the lumbar area
    fractures in the spine, hip, and front arm area.

TCM indications
Traditional Chinese practitioners believe osteoporosis is caused by one of more of the following elements:

1. **Deficiency of the liver and kidney.** The liver stores blood and dominates the tendons. The kidney stores *jing*, or *essence* and dominates the bones. Therefore, the condition of bone and tendons is directly related to the function of the liver and kidney.

2. **Kidney-jing deficiency.** Since the blood stored in the liver and the *jing* stored in the kidney can nourish both organs mutually, there is a TCM saying that *kidney and liver are derived from the same source*. So, the tendons and bones will fail to be nourished if there is a deficiency of blood or *jing*. The knee is the place where all the tendons gather. Deficiency of blood or *jing* will cause weakness in the knees and lower back pain.

3. **Qi and blood deficiency.** *Qi* and blood, as well as the kidney, nourish the brain. Deficiency in the *qi*, blood, liver and kidney leads to the brain being improperly nourished, therefore dizziness, *tinnitus* (ringing in the ears) and poor memory may occur. This deficiency may also cause premature loss of hair.

4. **Deficiency of yin/yang factor.** Kidney-*jing* not only includes *qi*, but also *yin and yang* aspects, therefore in deficiency of kidney *yin/yang* and/or *qi*, impotence is the main symptom, and lost sex drive.

When the body has *qi*, blood and kidney-*jing* deficiency, external pathogenic factors can easily invade. Weather or other changes can all make the person sick.

Case study:
A 50-year-old woman complained of night sweats, hot flushes, sharp pain in her shoulder area, lower back soreness. During sleep, her legs would cramp up two or three times a week. She experienced very poor memory, abdominal distention and water retention. Her periods had stopped a year previously. She had anxious feelings, palpitations in her chest, restless insomnia and complained of being overweight. Her tongue was slightly red with little coating, and a crack line in the center. Her pulse was thready and rapid.

TCM Diagnosis: Deficiency of yin, leading to osteoporosis.

The following are the Acupuncture points I used to treat her:
Upper limbs:
LI 15. jian yu (reducing method).
TW14. jian liao (reducing method).
Extra. jian Qian (even method).
LI10. Shou San Li (reinforcing method).

Lower limbs:
GB34. Yang Ling Quan (reducing method)
ST36. ZuSan Li (reinforcing method).
ST 41. Jie Xi (even method).
GB30. Huan Tiao (reducing method).

Points in the back:
Extra Hua Tuo Jia Ji (even method).

BL 23. Shen Shu (reinforcing method).
BL18. Gan Shu (reinforcing method).
Bl54. Zhi Bian (even method).

Within five treatments, the patient had no water retention, was sleeping better, and the leg cramps were relieved. In general she had more energy, and felt much less anxiety.

Class of Medicinal Herbs
Here are some herbs we can use for treatment of osteoporosis arthritis:

Shu Di Huang [Radix rhmanniae pracpparata]
Chuan Niu Xi [Radix cyathulae]
Du Zhong [Cortex eucommiae]
Dang Gui [Radix angelicae sinensis]
Huang Bai [Cortex phellodendri]
Huang Qi [Radix astragali membranacei]
Bu Gu Zhi [Fructus psoraleae]
Wu Wei Zi [Fructus schizandrae sinensis]
Gui Ban [Plastrum testudinis]

As I mentioned previously, osteoporosis is preventable, if you know how. Here are some guidelines to aid in prevention.

Prevention of Osteoporosis Arthritis
1. Eat bone soup or drink milk routinely. (Recipe for bone soup below)

2. Eat bean soup routinely.

3. Keep life simple. Avoid stress.

4. Watch your diet and be sure to get plenty of calcium. Proper consumption of nutritional foods and protein is needed. Vitamins are

vital to health and the prevention of osteoporosis. Calcium and phosphorous absorption in the body must be balanced, and vitamins speed up calcium absorption.

Foods rich in calcium include:
    shells of shrimp
    small fish
    soy products
    eggs
    kelp
    cabbage
    snails

Calcium in vegetables is often not properly absorbed by the human body, but adding vinegar during preparation can aid absorption. Vegetables like spinach and bamboo shoots contain oxalic acid in combination with calcium, and so don't need to be cooked with vinegar. Fruits like lemons, mandarin oranges and plums have citric acid, which performs the same function.

5. **Limit Alcohol.** Alcohol reduces calcium absorption, and lowers calcium concentration in the blood, so limit your consumption of alcoholic beverages.

6. **Limit Caffeine.** Coffee and tea cause calcium to be excreted out of the body in urine and feces. Drink these beverages moderately.

7. **Eat mushrooms.** Some fungi contain calcium and vitamin D, B1, B2 and phosphorous. These are good in the formation of bone matrix. "Monkey-head" mushrooms are particularly good, and grow naturally on walnut and birch trees. Fresh monkey-head mushrooms are as white as snow, and turn yellow or brown when dried. The monkey-head is delicious and good for the spleen, kidney and liver.

8. **Strengthen bones & tendons.** Exercise every day for 25-30 minutes. I recommend climbing stairs. Go up and down for 25 minutes daily. If we don't keep using the joints, we will lose function—that is a fact.

9. **Outdoor activities:** Sunlight can help produce vitamin D, which is vital for bone formation. Exercise stimulates skeletal growth, growth of bone mass, and slows down bone degeneration. Therefore, exercise prevents bone diseases when people grow older. Also it loosens up their joints and muscles and prevents fractures when they fall down. You can see that exercising outdoors in the daylight is beneficial.

10. **Avoid or limit use of certain medications.** Be aware of potential harm from some medications, such as corticosteroids, thyroid replacement drugs, heparin (a blood thinner), dilantin (which expands tubes that carry blood from the heart to cell tissues and organs). Ask for your doctor's consideration of the danger regarding osteoporosis.

11. Prevent or deal with *scoliosis* (spinal curvature). Often caused by bad posture, lack of exercise, or low dietary calcium, scoliosis is a concern when dealing with arthritis. Be sure to stretch your muscles in a balanced manner, use good posture all the time—that means when sitting, standing, exercising. Promote flexibility in all your joints.

12. Have a regular physical checkup. Use a standard method or procedure for bone density evaluation or a basis of comparison detected by plain radiographs, ultrasound, and x-ray densitometry to prevent problems.

Recipe for Bone Soup

An easy prevention for osteoporosis is to eat bone soup routinely—at least several times a week. Go to an Oriental market and get yourself a handful of ginger-root and also pick up the cheapest bones you can buy. These can be pig bones, chicken bones, cow/ox bones, and even fish bones (if you can stand the smell)—whichever you prefer.

When you return home, crush the ginger and put it in a large pot with the bones. Fill the pot with water and then boil for six to eight hours. If you wish to reduce the boiling time, simply add some vinegar. The vinegar will aid in extraction of the calcium.

Once you have boiled the soup, remove the ginger and bones and allow the soup to cool to room temperature before placing it in the refrigerator.

The next day when you open the container, you will see that the first layer in the soup is fat, and the second layer is a gelatin-like substance. Remove and discard the fat, and repack the gelatin and put it in the freezer—in an ice cube tray if you like. Whenever you cook anything that requires water, add the gelatin instead. Since the bone stuff came directly from animals, our body easily absorbs and uses it to supplement our bone marrow loss.

Chapter 11

Treating Osteoarthritis

How Natural Herbs and Acupuncture Can Heal Your Arthritis

Osteoarthritis is mainly characterized by pain, soreness, numbness and heaviness of the muscles and joints, with limitation of movement. The form of pain may vary from patient to patient. Very severe pain usually suggests intense causative factors or severe *qi* and blood stagnation. Although osteoarthritis is due to wind, cold and dampness, the cold factor predominates. The patient will have an aversion to cold and occasionally a slight fever.

TCM practitioners call osteoarthritis *Tong-Bi* or *Painful Bi* [painful syndrome]. This kind of *bi* [opponent] is characterized by heavy pain, very sharp or stabbing, and fixed, due to blood stagnation caused by cold. It is truly never a little pain. Sometimes the type of symptom changes. The quality of the pain changes: at times it can be sharp, other times there is soreness, at yet another time there is numbness. Later on there will be distending [expanding] pain. Different sensations occur, and sensitivity varies. Symptoms often appear abruptly. Sudden acute or paroxysmal pain occurs, and feels very "heavy." We call this *Bai Hu Feng*, which in English means *White Tiger Wind Disease*.

Sometimes we give different names to pain in varying locations. *Li Jie Feng* is periodic pain movement from one location or region to another. *He Xi Geng* or *Crane's Knee Wind*, refers to a red, swollen, painful knee. *Cao Xie Feng*, or *Straw Sandals' Wind*, refers to friction symptoms, like in the old days when people wore new straw shoes that caused skin to move back and forth with resulting abrasion and irritation.

External cold invasion of the individual causes a *yang* factor or defense energy restriction in the superficial layers of the body. The skin pores close and no sweat can escape. Consequently, the body must release fluids through the urine. Clear-colored urine is expelled frequently, in large quantities.

Besides lack of perspiration, chills are common, because the body is trying to maintain its normal temperature. The body's defense system, or *wei qi*, produces some warmth, so there can be some fever, but chills and feeling cold are predominant.

Osteoarthritis is a disease of long duration, and can occur repeatedly. It influences and affects the joint tissue, including cartilage breakdown and degeneration of the joint. There may be a combination of factors present. Probably every person past age 60 has osteoarthritis to some degree, but only a few actually have noticeable symptoms. It usually shows up at the site of an old injury.

According to the *Inner Classic* "Simple Questions," Chapter 44, serious injury to the body causes a syndrome involving weakness of the four limbs, skin, muscles, vessels, tendons, sinews and bones. Over a long period of time, our bodies will try to compensate for these old injuries, until there are new developments or the problem becomes more severe. Complex developments from old injuries can be osteoarthritis, arthritis, or hypertrophic arthritis. If the symptoms are bad enough to be noticed, then we will try to resolve the problem or seek medical care.

Treatment of Osteoarthritis

Treatment of osteoarthritis depends on the patient's reactions to wind-cold-damp, just as explained in the previous pages. In my clinical experience, osteoarthritis is generally cold predominant. The patient will feel stiffness and stickiness in the joint. In localized areas, the *qi* and blood will not be able to flow freely. If the patient is given heat or warmth it eases the pain, however, if coldness is applied, the pain will increase. The localized area feels cold with cold pain. In this case, treatment is to apply pungent, warm herbs to disperse the cold.

To warm the meridian, disperse the cold, and stop the pain, use:

> Aconitum radix
> Ephedra herba
> Astragalus radix
> Paeonia radix

to benefit the *qi* and nourish the blood. It is especially helpful to chronic sufferers and the elderly.

If the pain is extreme and does not subside, you may add:

> Clematis radix
> Curcuma rhizoma, and
> Rythrina cortex.

Case study:

A 60-year-old man suffered from hypertension, and had been under medication for five years. He came to my clinical complaining of extreme pain in his neck, a feeling of pressure in the head, dizziness, tinnitus, blurred vision, and dry eyes. He had been waking up four to five times during the night because his shoulders, back, knee joints, ankles and feet were hurting with sharp discomfort and extremely violent intense pain. It was difficult for him to perform normal daily physical motions. His face was red, as if he had sunburn. His tongue was red with no coating, with slight cracking on both sides. His pulse was wiry and thready.

Diagnosis: Deficiency of liver and kidney, causing liver *yang* rising.

The following are some of the acupuncture points and general method of treatment I used:

1) Even method, reinforcing method:
   LI 4, He Gu. TW4, Yang Qi, ST36, Zu San Li, LV3, Tai Chong, GB31, Feng Shi, GB34, Yang Ling Quan, TW5, Wai Guan.
2) Use of cupping and 7-star plum needles are combined to treat the affected part of the body. Make the area purplish, and then use cupping on top of it.
3) **Clinical experience points:**
   <u>Acute stage</u> Du 14. Da Zhui LI11. Qu Qi Du 12. Shen Zhu.
   <u>Chronic stage</u>: ST40. Feng Long. UB17 Ges Hu. SP10. Xue Hai.
   <u>Ah-shi points</u> [translated as *oh yes* points in English]: There are 12 regular meridians and 15 collateral channels running from the four limbs and circulating all over the body surface. These externally and internally related channels transport *qi*/blood to various tissues & organs, with recognized points between them. Ah-shi *points* are not recognized points, but when stimulated, work just as well as regular acupuncture points.
4) **Process for local areas:**
   Toe area: Ba feng, Liv.3 Tai Chong. Sp 3.Tai Bai.
   Ankle area: UB60 Kun Lun. Ki 3 .Tai xi. St41 Jie xi. Sp5 Shang Qiu.
   Knee area: Xi yian, St34. Liang Qiu UB40. Wei Zhong. GB34, Yang Ling Quan.
   Finger area: Ba xie. Si fong. LI 4,He Gu. TW5, Wai Guan. \ **Wrist area:** LI5.Yang Xi. SJ4.Yang Qi LI 4,He Gu. P7.Daling.
   Elbow area: LI11.Qu Qi. SI 8. Xiao Hai. SJ 10.Tian Jing.
   When using needles, even method is the best choice.

Gout

In my clinical studies I have much experience with gout, which is another form of osteoarthritis. Gout is caused by a defective uric acid metabolism. Urate crystals settle in various body tissues, including joints, triggering an inflammatory response. Fibrous tissue and giant cells develop, followed by local necrosis [death of the tissues].

Gout is classed as *primary* or *secondary*. In primary gout, hereditary factors cause uric acid overproduction and/or retention. Secondary gout results from use of certain drugs or appears as a complication of another disease or chronic kidney deficiency.

Normal uric acid levels in the body are 5mg/100ml, but in the gout patient are 8mg/100ml. Uric acid subsists in cartilage, joints, in the kidneys and tissue. If left untreated, it may lead to bony ankylosis, [abnormal union of bones in a joint], pathologic fracture, bone infarction [bone death], femoral head necrosis, urinary stones, renal disease, possibly leading to renal failure, cardiovascular lesions, cerebrovascular accident, coronary thrombosis, hypertension, infection with tophi rupture, or nerve entrapment. Take my advice and seek treatment if you have gout!

A painful episode of gout usually involves one joint—typically the great toe. Later acute attacks commonly affect several joints. Sometimes it will appear on the earlobes, fingers, hands, toes, ulnar forearm surface, and Achilles tendon. Renal function can also deteriorate.

Upon physical examination, the gout-affected joint is swollen, hot, dusky red or purple, is very sensitive to the touch, and has limited movement. Tophi [small stones, or crystals] may be noted, and sometimes fever and hypertension [high blood pressure]. The tophi are hard irregular yellow-white nodules, and they like to develop on the great toe and the earlobes, or other areas. Relatives of gout include any of several forms of infectious disease caused by *rickettsia* [infectious microorganisms], especially those transmitted by fleas, lice, or mites, and characterized generally by severe headache, sustained high fever, depression, delirium, and the eruption of red rashes on the skin.

In my opinion, the best choice of treatment for gout is immediate medical management. The doctor may order colchicine, indomethacin or phenylbutazone. The sooner therapy begins, the better the patient's response is.

Once the initial flare-up has subsided, the patient can be treated by eastern methods. This is the best way to solve the underlying problem.

Treatment for Gout

Practically, *Bi-syndrome* seldom appears by itself. Symptoms are very often mixed—therefore therapeutic rules need to be considered. Where do the symptoms occur? Do they originate or end in the roots, or in the branches? What should be treated first, or what should be treated second? Consideration must be given to all sides of the issue.

Knowing which pathogenic factors are most predominant is the key to treating gout. When pain has been present for a long time and joints show some deformity, we must not only circulate *qi* and blood or warm the meridians, but we must also adequately treat dampness, phlegm, and blood stagnation. For example, when gout resembles *scleroderma*, the TCM view is that the disease is due to blockage of blood in the skin. Therefore, promoting blood circulation is the key to successful treatment.

How should we treat the accumulation of phlegm and dampness in the meridians? For clinical symptoms of swelling, heaviness of body and head, lassitude, poor appetite, fullness of the chest and abdomen, loose stools, the TCM solution is to resolve the dampness and eliminate phlegm, circulate the blood and harmonize the meridians.

Sometimes painful symptoms can be due to deficient *qi* with blood stagnation. These symptoms are hard, rough or dry skin with a brown or purplish color, emaciation, dryness of the eyes and mouth. The TCM treatment is to *tonify qi* [restore energy] and nourish the blood, promote blood circulation and eliminate blood stasis.

Because the person with gout is not only suffering from *yang* deficiency with invasion by cold, he also has accumulation of *qi*, blood, phlegm and dampness in the meridians. In my clinical experience if this problem continues for a long time, it will lead to kidney, artery or vascular failure, heart diseases, or cerebral accident.

Medicinal Herb Use For Gout

In my experience I recommend the gout patient to see a western medical doctor for a better result. For *cold-Bi* syndrome, here are some herbs that can be used:

> Du Huo [Angelicae pubescentis]
> Han Fang Ji [Stephaniae tetrandrae]
> Qin Jiao [Radix fentianae macrophyllae]
> Wei Ling Xian [Radix clematidis sinensis]
> Qiang Huo [Rhizoma et Radix notopterygii]
> Cang Er Zi [Fructus xanthii]
> Xi Xin [Hera asari]
> Hai Tong Pi [Cortex erythrinae]

Prevention of Gout

In order to prevent an attack of gout, it is necessary to teach the patient about his disease.

Increase fluid intake to at least 2,000ml/day to prevent gallbladder, kidney or urinary bladder *calculi* [stones]. These stones are formed from minerals such as calcium, iron, potassium, sodium, zinc, or salts. Usually our body will produce, store or release stones by itself. According to *yin-yang* theory, when the body is out of balance, all normal properties change.

Learn about a proper diet. Because the body is developing uric acid, food is improperly absorbed or processed. Osteoarthritis, arthritis, and hypertrophic arthritis can be caused by weakness related to the stomach or intestines, or also the functions of the so-called "ductless glands," such as the thyroid, adrenal, or pituitary, and hormonal secretions. The body forms uric acid endogenously [from within], synthesizing the substance in gout, causing the patient to have disturbed purine metabolites—different from a normal person. It is essential to avoid foods high in purines to reduce metabolic stress. High-purine foods [those containing 100 to 1,000 mg of purine nitrogen/100g] include:

anchovies
bouillon
consommé
goose herring
mackerel
mincemeat
mussels
organ meats [brain, kidney, liver, heart]
partridge
roe
sardines
scallops
sweetbreads
yeast

Recommend limited intake of foods with moderate purine content [9 to 100mg of purine nitrogen/100g]. Such foods include:

asparagus
beans [dried]
fish
meat
mushrooms
peas [dried]
shellfish
spinach

An overweight patient should **lose weight slowly**. Fasting or crash dieting may cause an acute gout attack.

Avoid alcohol, or foods preserved in alcohol in order to maintain lower purine levels.

Maintain a regular routine. Stress and lack of sleep keep the body from regaining its balance.

Understand that infection, surgery, foreign protein therapy and radiation may also cause an acute gout episode.

If invasion by cold is most predominant, keep the body and meridians warm, and eat or drink appropriate warm foods.

If invasion by dampness and phlegm are most predominant, it is important to stay dry, and eat appropriate dry foods.

If *qi* and blood stagnation are most predominant, use TCM methods to try to soothe *qi* flow and nourish blood.

In treating gout, the whole idea is to find the causes, and remove them.

Chapter 12

Treating Rheumatoid arthritis

How Natural Herbs and Acupuncture Can Heal Your Arthritis

Rheumatoid arthritis is an *autoimmune* disease in which the body attacks its own healthy tissues. The membranes surrounding the joints become inflamed and release enzymes that can cause the surrounding cartilage and bone to deteriorate. The symptoms are chronic joint swelling and pain in fingers, hands, wrists, elbows, shoulders, knees, ankles, feet, etc. Over time the joints are less and less able to function, deformed and ultimately destroyed or immobile.

The ability to defend against microorganisms is called *immunity*. To state it more simply, the body can defend itself against invasion and colonization by foreign organisms. The word *immunity* is derived from the Latin *immuitas*, and in medicine, it denotes the "exemption from infection" that occurs under certain circumstances. Immunity to certain diseases means that a person has had that disease once and will not get it again.

In our daily lives we are exposed to many microorganisms: fine house dust, mites, pollen, fungal spores, feathers, animal dander and pet saliva, smoke, tobacco fumes, petrol fumes, unicellular prokaryotic microorganisms (schizomycetes). All of these can cause hypersensitivity and antigen production in the human body. Repeated exposure can cause the process of "clustering," a heavy thick grouping adhesion in our system, unquestionably causing disease.

Antigens stimulate the production of an antibody, which is a protein substance produced in the blood or tissues in response to a specific antigen, such as bacteria or toxins. Antibodies destroy or weaken bacteria and neutralize organic poisons, thus forming the basis of immunity. Antibody is a globulin formed in response to exposure to an antigen, an *immunoglobulin*.

The body's integrated system of organs, tissues and cells—or the lymphoid system—is able to neutralize potentially pathogenic organisms. The lymphoid system, or immune system, is defense against microorganisms entering the body. When we enter a foreign country, we are obligated to produce an official permit to travel into that country. The border guards recognize the permit. In the same way, the lymphoid system can recognize what organisms are permitted to travel into the body. The immune system is able to differentiate between those elements that are foreign to the body and those existing.

An important property of the immune system *immunologic* memory is that when a foreign molecule is encountered, the immune system responds more vigorously and rapidly than it did the first time. Derangement of the immune system may result in hypersensitivity, autoimmune disorders, *immunodeficiency* diseases, and tumor diseases.

If the body's immune system is weak, invasion by microorganisms is possible. The security guards don't recognize the danger, because they are sick, or tired. The body doesn't recognize the need to fight off the invasion. Or, conversely, the security guards react to every perceived threat, instead of just the recognized dangers. They shoot every person who comes to the border.

As mentioned, rheumatoid arthritis is an inflammatory disease resulting from the body's over-or under-reactive immune system. Why do we believe it is an autoimmune disorder? The medical profession tells us:

1. The C-reactive protein in the immunoglobulin fraction is increased in the serum.
2. Denatured immunoglobulin is also increased in the serum of these patients. Therefore, IgG and anti-IgG antibodies are deposited in the joints, their presence eliciting the inflammatory reactions leading to swelling and pain in the joints.

It is known that an immune system that is too weak can cause the body to become over-reactive. In the same way, an extremely strong immune system will cause the body to become over-reactive. Keeping the body harmonized is the key to treating rheumatoid arthritis.

Clinical symptoms and signs:
1. **Pain.** The most common symptom of RA, pain can be divided into the *excessive* and/or *deficient* type. According to TCM, it can be excessive due to obstruction, or deficient due to poor nourishment.

2. **Limitation of flexion and extension.** Morning stiffness is especially common with rheumatoid arthritis, plus mechanical physical difficulty with joints, and even includes tissues, muscles, tendons and bones.

3. **Swelling and deformity of joints.** Joints, tissues—the whole body—all need to be properly nourished by *qi*, blood, and body fluids. Invasion by external pathogenic factors causes stagnation of *qi*, blood, and body fluids. The long-term accumulation of wind, cold, and damp encourages the formation of phlegm and blood stagnation in the joints. Malnutrition increases, the joints fail to be nourished, and the joints become progressively deformed.

4. **Thickness and discoloration of the skin.** Chronic swelling of the skin will cause thickness, induce stagnation of *qi* and blood locally, so hardness and discoloration occur, or nodules may appear under the skin.

Clinically, the signs and symptoms of RA are very much the same as other types of arthritis, however is often noted that people with rheumatoid arthritis are extremely sensitive to weather changes.

This is where differentiation is valuable. Knowing the differences between osteoporosis, osteoarthritis, and rheumatoid arthritis becomes very important because sometimes it is very difficult to separate the symptoms, and the result of treatment will be poor if based on the wrong premise.

> Treatment of rheumatoid arthritis is:
> Acupuncture
> Acupuncture
> Acupuncture

Acupuncture can restore the body's harmony, invigorate the blood circulation and calm the spirit.

TCM indications

Stagnation and blockage in the meridians form the *Bi-syndromes*. However, stagnation can be caused by different factors, such as wind, cold, damp, heat, phlegm and blood stasis. Depending on which is the predominant factor, one can choose the proper therapeutic method of treatment.

1. Invasion by wind, cold, damp into meridians.
2. Obstruction of *qi* and blood.

Case study:

A 45-year-old woman had been suffering from joint pain for 10 years. For treatment, she was taking daily one *Ketoprofen* (NSAID), which would commonly take care of the problem. Lately it would take longer to work, and sometimes she still felt tension, numbness, heaviness, or would experience a condition that felt like the insides of her joints were boiling.

Her tongue was slightly pale with a red tip, swollen and puffy with teeth marks, and had a thin white, greasy, sticky coating. Pulse was weak and thready without strength.

Diagnosis: Rheumatoid Arthritis—wind, cold, dampness invading the body causing obstruction and stagnation of blood.

The following are some of the acupuncture points, herbs and general method I used to assist her.

Acupuncture points:
To circulate through the channels and harmonize the tendons:
GB34. Yang Ling Quan GB37, Guangg Ming.
GB40. Qiu Xu. LV3. Tai Chong.
LV5. Li Gou. LV8. QuQuan.
SP6. San Yin JIao.

Method: all even method. Moxibustion is applicable, except in cases of heat symptoms.

To eliminate phlegm and remove blood stasis:
LI .4, He Gu. LI.11.Qu Qi
LI10. Shou San Li. TW 6. ZhiGou
CV12.Zhong Wan. ST.40.Feng Long.
SP.10. Xue Hai. SP6. San Yin JIao.

Method: reducing method. Moxibustion may be applied if there are no heat signs.

Class of Medicinal Herbs Used:
To circulate through the channels and harmonize the tendons:
Treat chronic *Bi-syndromes* which are causing channel and tendon block-

age. Symptoms and signs are severe pain, stiffness and deformity of joints, difficulty in flexion and extension.

Di Long [Lumbricus]
Quan Xie [Scorpio]
Chuan Shan Jia [Squama manitis]
Shui Zhi [Hirudo seu whitmania]
Wu Gong [Scolopendra]
Lu Feng Fang [Nidus vespae]
Bai Hua She [Agkistrodon seu bungaruss]
Wu Shao She [Zaocys]

To eliminate phlegm and remove blood stasis:
Treat invasion by dampness, and blockage of meridians due to a mixture of phlegm accumulation and blood stasis in the joints.

Zhu Li. [Succus bambusae]
Sheng jiang Zhi [Rhizoma zingiberis recens melle tostum]
Ban Zia [Rhizoma pinelliae praeparatum]
Bai jie Zi [Semen sinapis albae]
Fu Ling [Sclerotium poriae albae]
Dan Nan Xing [Rhizoma arisaematis cum felle bovis]
Bai Jiang can. [Bombyx barryticatus]
Ju Luo [Fasciculus vascularis aurantii]
Si Gua Luo [Fasciculus vascularis luffae]
Chuan AXiong [Rhizoma ligustici]
Ru Xiang [Resina olibani]
Mo Yao [Resina myrrhae]
Hong Hua [Flos carthami]
Di Long [Lumbricus]
Chuan Shan Jia [Squama manitis]

Result: After lengthy treatment twice a week for more than two years, the patient feels good with little joint pain. An added benefit is that she looks much younger, is happy and enjoys life.

Prevention of Rheumatoid Arthritis

Today in China, it has been proved repeatedly by experience and experimentation that acupuncture and herbs have a strengthening effect on the body's resistance and can prevent rheumatoid arthritis, as well as certain other acute chronic inflammatory conditions. Experimental research has shown that during acupuncture treatments the immunological system is strengthened, immunological functions are enhanced, metabolism is regulated, and normal organ function is restored.

Acupuncture and herbs have analgesic and organ function regulation effects, and working together with the immunologic effect will enhance the resistance of the body. The anti-inflammatory effect of acupuncture owes to the combined function of the autonomic nervous system, blood circulation, cellular activity and hormonal activities of endocrine glands. The autonomic nervous system is the system of nerves and ganglia in the blood vessels, heart, smooth muscles, viscera and glands and controls their involuntary functions.

1. **Keeping balanced** is the best way to prevent RA, but in today's society this is almost impossible. The person who suffers from this disease, or knows he may inherit it genetically from his parents, should give up money and time. Go for routine acupuncture in order to take care of rheumatoid arthritis. By the way, I have very good results in treating this disease.

2. **Be confident.** Thinking positive is a must to prevent and treat RA.

3. **Try to avoid direct exposure to sunlight.** If you cannot avoid it, use sunscreen lotion, an umbrella, a big hat, long shirt and pants. Don't apply sun reflection chemicals (sun block).

4. **Avoid overwork, exhaustion, pregnancy.**

5. **Take care of damaged kidneys first.** If a person knows his kidneys don't function properly or if they have been damaged, he needs to take care of this first, otherwise an attack of rheumatoid arthritis will be more severe.

6. **Avoid common infections**, such as the common cold and other infections.

7. **Exercise.** Improvement in body strength requires everyday physical or mental exertion. One must work daily to develop or maintain fitness.

8. **Nutrition.** Nourishing or being nourished is a key issue of growth and replacement. Proper food intake is needed, as well as supplementation with various natural plants and vitamins.

9. **TCM.** The results are slow in coming, but you must be patient and try to understand how TCM works. It will take care of you.

Herbs that will help include:
Radix et rhizoma notopterygii
Radix angelicae pubescentis
Rhizoma et radix lingustici
Radix ledebouriellae divaricatae
Radix glycyrrhizae uralensis
Radix ligustici chuanxiong
Fructus viticis

These herbs can expel wind-dampness, arrest pain and relieve the exterior. The results I have seen have been good.

Chapter 13

Treating Rheumatic Arthritis

How Natural Herbs and Acupuncture Can Heal Your Arthritis

Rheumatic arthritis usually occurs as a result of bacterial infection. Sometimes it happens due to drug abuse, diabetes *mellitus*, sickle-cell anemia or chronic infection, but most commonly it is caused by *staphylococcus*. *Auras* organisms, various fungi, and viruses can also be to blame.

Whatever the cause, inflammation can spread through the fibrous connective layer of tissue covering the bones, through the outer layer, or the cortex, and penetrate deep inside the bone. Rheumatic arthritis is extremely painful, and can cause the body to be vulnerable to further risk.

Symptoms include sudden high fever, accompanied by local inflammation, redness around the joint, heat, pain and swelling. Rest doesn't relieve the pain. The range of joint motion is limited, and moving increases discomfort. The patient refuses to be touched or palpated. If such symptoms exist, take heed of my advice: Go immediately to a medical institution and have it checked out.

Now remember that acute rheumatic arthritis always starts with fever. Fever can be high, moderate, or even low, and comes with profuse sweating. The heartbeat increases, joint pain is severe and moves from place to place. Some of the joint pains are fixed in one location, like at the knee, ankle, shoulder, and hip area, and are red, swollen, hot, and painful. The inflammation usually does not deform the joints. In some cases the blood vessels, the kidneys, the nerves and other organs of the body are involved.

The number one concern with rheumatic arthritis is that it will lead to heart disease. Once rheumatic arthritis is established in the body, the resulting inflammation can begin to affect all its systems, including the cardiovascular system. This is the transportation system of the body, and consists of the arteries, capillaries, and veins—which form a closed loop—and the lymphatic network. The heart brings life-supporting oxygen and nutrients to cells, removes metabolic waste products, and brings hormones from one part of the body to another. Diseases of the heart relative to arthritis may either be congenital, inflammatory, degenerative, or due to tumors.

Valvular Disease

Rheumatic fever is an inflammatory disease that occurs in the body after a group A *beta-streptococcal* infection has been present. It affects all the body's systems. Symptoms include fever, migratory joint pain, swelling, redness, "leaking" of the heart's valves, skin lesions, inflammation, nodules under the skin, involuntary movement or jerking, elevated white blood count. Repeated infection and improperly treated rheumatic fever may cause the heart to accumulate valvular lesions, such as *stenosis*—the narrowing of the *mitral* and *aortic* valve opening—and regurgitation incompetence of the valve. This may result in interfered *hemodynamics* (circulation of the blood), *myocardial* (heart) damage, blood clot formation, and could lead to heart failure.

Simply stated, just as in a car engine if a valve is not sealed properly, oil or other fluids will leak and cause smoking. Disease of the valve located at both sides of the heart pump valve will not allow the artery or vein to fold or close suitably, and fit properly. The fluid (blood) cannot be sealed inside, as it should be.

TCM indications

Vascular or blood vessel problems belong to *Bi* symptoms: stagnation of blood blocking the vessels and causing pain. Pains are stabbing, aggravated at night, and relate to muscles and joints. Other symptoms are an uneasy feeling, uncomfortable sensation, especially in the left side chest area, feeling of distress, anxiety, sudden shortness of breath, dryness of the upper throat, frequent belching, a burning sensation of the skin. There may be red or purplish spots in or under the skin that look like rash eruptions.

Rheumatic arthritis can come suddenly and it will occur over and over again, becoming a chronic disease. Never underestimate it—take it seriously and immediately go to the hospital for proper treatment.

TCM Treatment of Rheumatic Arthritis

After the medical establishment has dealt with the acute symptoms, we must look for a solution to the root of the problems.

Mostly symptoms of rheumatic arthritis are mixed, other than wind, cold, and dampness. *Bi*-symptoms of heat signs are predominant.

Case study:

A 32-year-old overweight woman went to the hospital for treatment of severe pain and rigidity in her neck. She had itchy bumps on her skin, filled with fluid, which turned to pustules. Since her return from hospital a week previously, she felt extremely tired and her limbs were heavy and achy. She was hot and thirsty with a continuous sticky feeling in her mouth. She also had some abdominal pain and loose stools. Due to dampness and heat, her pulse was slippery and rapid. Her tongue was red and swollen with a thick sticky yellow coating.

Diagnosis: Infection. Retention of dampness, heat in the large intestine.

The following are some of the acupuncture points, herbs and general methods I used to assist her:

To clear the heat and remove toxins:
Acupuncture points:
LI4. He Gu. LI11. Qu Qi.
GB20. Feng Qi. TW5. Wai Guan.
ST44. Nei Ting. LV2.Xing Jia
BL17. Ge Shu.

Method: Reducing method. Do not use moxibustion in this case.

Class of Medicinal Herbs to use:
Besides acupuncture and herbal treatment, dietetic measures also are very important in dealing with vascular *Bi*-symptoms.

Tu Fu Ling [Rhizoma smilacis glabrae]
Shui Niu Jiao [Cornu bubali]
Sheng Di Huang [Radix rehmammiae recens]
Qi Shao Yao [Radix paeoniae rubrae]
Mu Dan Pi [Cortex moutan radicis]
Ren Dong Teng [Caulis seu ramus lonicerae]
Yi Yi Ren [Semen coicis]
Huang Bai [Cortex phellodendri]
Zhi Mu [Rhizoma anemarrhenae]
Jin Yin Hua. [Flos lonicerae]
Lian Qiao [Fructus forsythiae]
Pu Gjong Ying [Herba taraxaci cum radice]
Zi Hua Di Ding [Herba violae cum radices]
Di Gu Pi [Cortex lycii radicis]

Results: After one treatment, the woman felt much better. The pus and diarrhea disappeared.

Prevention of Rheumatic Arthritis

1. Improve your body's strength through daily exercise. Like the old Chinese saying, *Zang qi strong, then evil qi never wins.*

2. Keep warm and avoid cold, because rheumatic arthritis starts from wind, cold and dampness. Avoid sleeping or living in damp or moist places.

3. Keep your immune system strong, and your yin-yang in balance. Avoid beta-streptococcal infections by staying out of public areas as much as possible. A strong immune system can exempt you from acute contagious viral infections and fever, chills, muscular pain, and prostration.

4. Acupuncture and herbs can help to improve the body's defenses against attack.

5. Get plenty of rest and drink sufficient water.

Chapter 14

Treating Traumatized Arthritis

How Natural Herbs and Acupuncture Can Heal Your Arthritis

The traditional Chinese physician believes that arthritis is caused by pathogenic factors invading the body. These outside pathogenic factors are: wind, cold, damp, heat, summer heat and dryness. Among these six pathogenic factors wind, cold and dampness are the most common causes of joint "sickness."

Why do pathogenic factors invade our joints? As we already discussed, these factors are originally normal weather conditions. When human immune systems are weak, or *Zang Qi is insufficient*, then microorganisms can invade the body and cause illness.

However, the causes of traumatized arthritis are a little different than pathogenic factors invading. Traumatized arthritis occurs when the body suffers from internal and/or external shock. It relates to the body's mechanics, as distinguished from the mind or spirit. It is characterized by violence.

Common disorders from spasm, cramp, bruises, or strains often cause the ligaments and other soft tissue to be damaged. If proper treatment is not given when the initial injury occurs, these factors can become acute infectious or chronic traumatized arthritis. Some of these common disorders are:

1. **Bursitis:** Inflammation of the bursa, a sac between tendon and bone, caused by irritation, overuse, or repeated minor trauma, especially in the shoulder, elbow, or knee joint.

2. **Sprains:** When a joint is forced past the limits of its normal movement. Hemorrhages and tears in the fibers of the ligament can occur and painful wrenching or deep emotional pain can result.

3. **Ligament damage:** Can occur when a joint is moved past its normal range of movement, or degenerates due to changes caused by age or lack of use. Ligament damage caused by traumatic forces can inflame all the neighboring structures as well.

4. **Strains:** When excessive pressure or stress happens to the body or mind, muscles, nerves, or tendon tissues are stretched tight or torn. A sudden sharp twist or turn causing a complex of damage is called a strain.

5. **Cramp:** The muscle or muscles suddenly contract. A sudden, involuntary, spasmodic muscular contraction, such as what happens in the uterus or abdomen due to menstruation or labor, can also occur in the lower back, leg, thigh, or shoulder, and causes severe pain.

6. **Spasm:** A spasm is a sudden, involuntary contraction of a muscle or group of muscles, or a sudden burst of energy, activity, or emotion. Spasms can be acute or chronic. The underlying cause of acute spasms can be easily solved. Chronic spasms sometimes change muscle tissue or cause the formation of excessive fibrous tissue, making the muscle drier and stringy.

7. **Inflammation:** Inflammation occurs when the body protects itself after injury or disease. When tissue is damaged, the white blood cells,

which are our military force, race to the scene of the crime and produce substances called *prostaglandins* and *leukotrienes*. This brings on a multitude of biochemical reactions including inflammation.

8. **Clinical Symptoms and Signs of Traumatized Arthritis**
Traumatized arthritis can be acute or chronic. Acute traumatized arthritis usually arises from:

a) An unexpected, undesirable event, or
b) An unfortunate incident due to being in the wrong place at the wrong time, or commencing activities without sufficient preparation. (For example, warm up, stretch, before jogging, etc.)

a) You may differentiate between the two as: being from trauma caused by outside factors, or that caused by inside factors, such as those relating to organs such as the heart, lung, brain, etc.
b) Chronic traumatized arthritis usually encompasses more than one cause, sometimes including internal organ involvement and complications. But generally speaking, traumatized arthritis is illness without a systemic cause. Pain can be severe with tenderness and swelling, and lack of mobility. Sometimes it is characterized by stabbing pain, tiredness, dizziness, purplish color of the muscles, and swelling around the wound.

Old injuries can become inflamed again, usually when one is overworked, exhausted, and unable to concentrate. The best way to avoid the re-inflammation of an old injury is to avoid exhaustion, physical overwork, and mental strain.

TCM Indications:
External stagnation of *Qi* and blood.
Deficiency of kidney-*jing*.

Treatment of Traumatized Arthritis
Use careful palpation to make sure there are no broken bones, fragments, open wound or protrusion. If there are any of these, send the patient to an institution that provides medical, surgical, or physical care right away. If there is no sign of the above symptoms, use TCM methods to:

1. Eliminate blood stagnation. Remove the blockages to allow the blood to flow freely.
2. Circulate the *Qi* and blood.
3. Consolidate, or strengthen, the bones.

We want to stop the pain, remove the obstruction and invigorate the blood circulation. In other words, we want to end the pain and allow the injured area to heal quickly. Many people use cold or hot pads or use pain relievers. In my opinion, and through my clinical experience, these methods are not the best ways to treat traumatized arthritis.

My recommendation in the case of traumatized arthritis is acupuncture treatment. During treatment, it is best to massage and relax the side of the body opposite to that of the injured one. For example, if you had injured your right ankle, you would massage your left wrist first (especially the tender areas around your wrist).

Acupuncture points
1. Use acupuncture at Ear points, or *Auricular* points. When body disorders occur, a reaction will appear at the corresponding area of the ears, such as tenderness, numbness, structural changes, and discoloration. Using acupuncture in these sensitive ear points can treat or prevent diseases.

2. Sprains or strains have more than one meridian involved; therefore it
    is often helpful to use acupuncture at local and *Ah-shi* points. *Ah-shi*
    points are tender and sensitive areas or points that are not in the
    regular meridian path, and can be stimulated to relieve the problem.

3. Rub ginger-root and natural raw vinegar on the affected area, and
    strike lightly with plum-blossom needle or seven-star hammer. (A
    seven-star hammer is made of five to seven stainless steel needles
    inlaid onto the end of a handle. It pricks the skin superficially by
    tapping, to promote the smooth flow of *qi* and regulate the energy.) Or
    strike at the following points:

    GB 34. Yang Ling Quan. GB37. Guang Ming.
    GB40. Qiu Xu. LV 3.Tai Chong.
    LV5. Li Gou. LV8.Qu Quan.
    Sp6. San Yin Jiao.

Method: even method. Moxibustion is applicable, except in case
where heat is present.

For external stagnation of Qi and blood:
1. Rest. If heat and swelling are predominant, clear the heat and swell-
    ing by using TCM methods.

2. If sprain or strain are located in an extremity, such as in a limb or the
    foot, treat the opposite and across side first. For example, in the case
    of injured right medial side of foot, treat left lateral side hand.

Case study:
A 35-year-old woman had been suffering from sprain and strain. Her
feet and ankles were swollen and painful. She also suffered from lower
backache as well. Her tongue was pale, purple with a thin coating. Her
pulse was deep and weak, and occasionally choppy and uneven.

Diagnosis: Traumatized arthritis due to deficiency, cold and retention of *qi* and blood.

The following are some of the acupuncture points, herbs and general method I used to assist her:

Acupuncture points:
GB 34. Yang Ling Quan. GB37. Guang Ming.
GB40. Qiu Xu. LV 3. Tai Chong.
LV5. Li Gou. LV8. Qu Quan.
Sp6. San Yin Jiao.

Method: even method. Moxibustion is applicable, except in case of Heat.

Class of Medicinal Herbs to Use:
To circulate the meridians and harmonize the tendons:
Di Long [Lumbricus]
Quan Xie [Scorpio]
Chuan Shan Jia [Squama manitis]
Wu Gong [Scolopendra]
Lu Feng Fang [Nidus vespae]
Bai Hua She [Agkistrodon seu bungarus]
Wu Shao She [Zaocys eupolyphaga seu opisthoplatia]

To warm the kidney and benefit the bones:
Zhi Fu Zi [Radix aconiti lateralis praeparata]
Rou Gui [Cortex cinnamomi]
Suo Uang [Herba cynomorii]
Ba Ji Tian [Radix morinadae officinalis]
Sang Ji Sheng [Ramulus loranthi]
Xu Duan [Radix dipsaci]
Du Zhong [Cortex eucommiac]
Bu Gu Zhi [Fructus psoraleae]
Huai Niu Xi [Radix achyranthis bidentatae]
Shu Di Huang [Radix rehmanniae praepparata]
Tu Bie Chong [Eupolyphaga seu opisthoplatia]

Results: After five treatments, the patient had no swelling or pain.

As I said, the best method of treatment for traumatized arthritis is acupuncture, however, there are times when we do not have acupuncturists at hand and so we must use some ancient and not-so-ancient Chinese recipes.

Using hot water, as hot as you can stand, soak the area for 20 to 25 minutes while massaging it. You may also sprinkle a handful of salt into the water. If possible you should soak the joint in vinegar or cover the injury in a vinegar-soaked cloth.

Try to find this special point on the body. In my clinical experience, even without a needle you can very effectively relieve the injury, or at least make it less unpleasant. Find the point as described below, and use your hand or thumb to massage there deeply and vigorously.

When elbow is flexed slightly, hold the fist with the palm face down. The point is three fingers from your elbow crease on the top of the arm. This area is always somewhat sore or tender.

Never apply ice, or soak the injury in cold water. Absorb hot water instead. You should seek to reduce the swelling and inflammation. If there is no broken skin or open wound, soak in hot water, as hot as you can take it, with a cup of Epsom salt and 75% rubbing alcohol for 20-25 minutes. Repeat this process as frequently as possible (6-7 times a day), and you will recover much faster. I have very good results with this method.

I had a patient with a sprained ankle. After acupuncture and this soaking process above, he was able to walk again the next day.

Let me explain why the use of ice is not recommended. While the application of ice or cold will make the area feel better faster, it also stops the circulation of blood or fluids rushing to repair your injury. Ice causes these fluids to "freeze" or change shape. The capillaries contract, and the blood that is frozen out of the capillary or out of the artery never returns to its normal fluid state. The body cannot clean up these fragments completely. In the long term, the area will not heal properly, or takes longer to repair, because circulation is not comprehensive. The environment in the local area is never the same. The application of heat, while maybe uncomfortable, promotes the circulation of these healing fluids, causing faster repair.

Over-usage or over-damage, such as experienced by athletes who use the same joints over and over again for a long period of time, can easily cause local pain and swelling. It is necessary to seek medical attention as soon as possible in these cases. Before the physician arrives, the athlete can use the process stated above.

Go to an herbalist and acquire 30g of *Radix et rizoma rhei* and 30g of *Mirabilitum*. Take the herbs home, cover with water, and boil for 10 to 20 minutes. Cool to a temperature that you feel is the maximum heat that you can take. Soak the injured area for 20 to 25 minutes. Repeat this procedure as often as possible.

*Herbs to Use to Bathe or Soak traumatized area:
Cao Wu [Wild aconite root-processed]
Chuan Wu [Sichuan aconite root-processed]
Dang Gui [Angelicae radix]
Du Huo [Pubescent angelica root]
Hong Hua [Carthamus]
Lu Lu Tong [Liquidambar]
Mo Yao [Myrrha]
Mu Dan Pi [Moutan radicis cortex]
Mu Gua [Chaenomeles]
Qiang Huo [Notopterugium root]
Rou Gui [Cinnamon bark]
Ru Xiang [Mastic]
Shen Jin Cao [Buck grass]
Yi Mu Cao [Leonurus]

*Statistics show that total dosage weight of herbs must be more than 1000 grams or 1kg to be effective. Add water and heat to boiling.

Prevention of Traumatized Arthritis

According to "*Huang Di Nei Jing*" or *Yellow Emperor's Internal Classic*, Chapter 44, *Simple Questions*, the Trauma Syndrome is a condition of weakness in the four limbs, skin, muscles, vessels, tendons, sinews and bones. To avoid the occurrence of traumatized arthritis, follow these guidelines.

1. **Avoid damp heat**, because it dries up the body's fluids. Injury is caused to skin, muscles, vessels, tendons, sinews and bones over a long period of time when there is exposure to damp heat. Without proper nourishment, the components mentioned become deficient, leading to weakness. This deficiency happens gradually, and paves the way for accidents to occur, damaging the affected parts before any pain is noticed.

2. **Try to maintain all your functions in harmony.** According to TCM's Five Element Theory (circulation, promotion and generation of wood, fire, earth, metal and water), the essential principle of preventing traumatized arthritis is to be sure the body is harmonized. From the internal organs' condition to a stable mental or psychological state and emotional stability—all must be balanced to prevent a deficiency of skin, muscles, vessels, tendons, sinews and bones.

3. **Avoid invasion of cold dampness.** Cold dampness manifests in the body as feeling cold, a heavy sensation in the legs, nausea, poor appetite, edema, hemorrhage, bloody stools, a craving for sweets. If you have some body manifestation or the presence of cold and dampness is noticed, try to resolve the problem as soon as possible.

4. **Avoid invasion of wind heat.** Because wind speeds up heat and becomes fire, it will rapidly dry up the body fluids and yin factor. The drying up of fluids leads to malnourishment of skin, muscles, vessels, tendons, sinews and bones. Therefore, keep it from happening by keeping cool and drinking plenty of fluids.

5. **Consolidate the bones**—keep the bone structure strong. The kidney organs store kidney essence, which is responsible for reproduction, growth and development, and marrow production. Kidney essence governs the bones. Therefore, excessive sexual activity and overwork without proper rest will weaken bones and sinews, leading to the occurrence of traumatized arthritis.

6. **Watch your diet.** You are what you are eating, so make sure your body is able to properly consume food. Intake of too much dairy food, irregular eating habits, overeating, consumption of alcohol, especially hard liquor, use of drugs and tobacco will cause weakening of muscles.

7. **Exercise daily.** Walking, stooping, gathering, gardening, hunting, hiking, stair-climbing—all can prevent atrophy in the muscles, im-

prove strength or tone muscles, reduce bone and cartilage thinning and softening.

If we don't keep using the joints, we will lose function—that is a fact. Exercise strengthens the bones and their supporting structures— muscles, tendons, ligaments—and increases range of motion, shock absorption, and flexibility of the joints. Exercise improves the body's physical capabilities, prevents joint deformities, reduces stress, promotes relaxation. It also improves body composition, and increases the immune system resistance to disease.

The activity you choose should cause the heart to pump and circulate blood through all your bodily vessels. Running or stair climbing is excellent. Stretching exercises such as yoga and *qi kong* and aerobic conditioning are highly recommended and important to improve body flexibility and avoid certain injuries. The type of exercise you do doesn't really matter, as long as you have a pleasurable and satisfactory time and are able to do it without disadvantage or risk to your normal healthy condition. Try to maintain or develop body fitness.

8. **Breathe.** Learn to inhale and exhale fully, especially in a natural and unlabored manner.

9. **Exercise your mind daily**. Too much sitting around can deeply affect the mind and emotions. Practice meditation, prayer or other process of spiritual activity. Practice *qi kong*, or yoga—any system of exercises balanced so as to promote control of the body and mind. Learning to be flexible and responsive to change is key to prevention of traumatized arthritis.

Chapter 15

Case Studies

Case Study 1

A 36-year-old woman was involved in a very emotional family fight last night. This morning she woke up and found both her feet were very sore, and not able to support her body. Her family immediately sent her to the hospital to see a neurologist. A routine check was performed. Knee reflexor, all physical exams were normal. After several hours of observation, the hospital released the patient.

Someone recommended checking with an Oriental physician to try to find something. Through TCM examination it was found that her tongue coating was yellowish, thick and greasy. Her pulse was slippery and rapid. She had scant and dark yellow urine. Diagnosis was Dampness Heat accumulation.

Diagnosis: Because of the anger and emotion of the previous night, the cause was determined to be Liver Fire. Liver Fire is a branch of Dampness Heat. Dampness Heat is the root of the problem.

Treatment: In order to take care of this problem we have to clear the Liver Fire, which will take care of the Dampness Heat.

Herbs used:
Long dan tsao
Huang chin
Huang bao
Zhe she
Che chen zhi
Tsang zu
Niu che
Mu tong

Case Study 2

A woman, 39 years old, came with both feet and lower extremities swollen, complaining of sharp pain, especially near the gastrocnemial muscle (lower leg) area. For the past month she had been having difficulty walking. Her personal description of the pain was "heat penetrating running up from the foot all the way to the side." She also had a cough, palpitations, and insomnia. The previous couple of days, she had been coughing up a little bit of blood with mucus, and she had an afternoon fever. In addition, she had scant urine, constipation, rapid pulse, and a red tongue with yellow coating.

Diagnosis: According to the *Inner Classic*, every time you see the top of a patient's foot swollen, the cause is fire.

Treatment: The solution is to clear the heat and harmonize the lower meridian.

Herbs used:
San bai pi
Di gu pi
Sen shi gao
Tsao dan pi
Tse shao

Len shin
Bai he
Shin ren
Zhe mu
Shen ru gen
Gan tsao

Recovery:

In both of these cases, after 7-10 treatments, both patients recovered sufficiently to be somewhat mobile. On a scale of 0-10, where 0 means lost function, and 10 fully able to walk, each of their recoveries can be judged as "5."

These two cases have something in common. Both patients cannot walk and are in pain. In the western point of view their symptoms belong to a disease called multiple sclerosis. Multiple sclerosis is the most common neurological disease. Its pathology consists of partial destruction of myelin sheaths along the spinal cord, brain, and optic nerves. The lesions are dissimilate at intervals and the many various symptoms depend on the locations of the lesions. Because the lesions can partially heal, the disease goes through characteristic phases of remission and relapse.

Why do I mention this disease in connection with arthritis? Many kinds of arthritis can lead to MS. According to western medical philosophy, the causes of MS are unknown. In TCM, we believe it can be caused by a combination of reasons, one being complications from the long-term use of pharmaceutical drugs. Since the current accepted treatment of arthritis involves the long-term use of pharmaceuticals, a consequent development can be MS syndrome.

Over time, drug use can affect the body's inner arteries, making them hollow. The structures lose strength, and are unable to support the body.

147

In young people the first presented symptom is usually *retrobulbar* (a blocked tube or passageway, that becomes abnormally enlarged or dilated), while in old people it is weakness in the leg. This disease is characterized by many different symptoms according to the lesions in the myelin sheaths. These symptoms include blurred vision, weakness and heaviness in one or both legs, jerking of the legs, double vision, vertigo, vomiting, uncoordination, a feeling in the arms and legs of suffering an electric shock, numbness and tingling of limbs, urgency or hesitation of urination, impotency.

In progressive degeneration of the myelin sheaths, there is an increased uncoordination and weakness of the legs and arms. In the late stage there is complete paralysis of the spastic type, together with urinary incontinence and brain disturbance with involuntary shaking, jerking of the legs or arms, weakened nerves and muscles, electrical shocks, tingling, cold, slight vibration, or rapid, tremulous movement.

Multiple Sclerosis or dermatomyositis or so-called polymyositis—to me they are all the same—are similar to muscle, tissue, and tendon problems. The Traditional Chinese Medical treatment would segregate it into two types: acute syndrome and chronic syndrome. If it is an acute syndrome the treatment and principle is mainly to clear the heat, detoxify, promote dampness, reduce swelling.

Usually we use two main prescriptions:
Yin Chen hao tang and *bei shei shen shi tang* in a combination together.
Yin chin hao tang is made with:
  Yin chin
  Zhe zhi
  Da Huang

Bei shei shen shi is made with the following ingredients:
  Bei shei
  Yi yi ren
  Huang bua

Tse hu ling
Mu dan pei
Zhe she
Tong tsao

For chronic diseases the cause is gradual and the disease is more moderate, so therefore the treatment method is to nourish the blood, benefit the *qi*, tonify/supplement the spleen and kidneys.

Generally prescribed: *gui pi tang, wu zhong yi qi wan*, or *shi chun da bu tang*.

Gui pi tang is created with the following ingredients:
Bai zsu
Fu shen
Huang chee
Long yen ro
Suan zha ren
Dan shen
Mu shang
Zhi gang tsao
Yuan zhi
Dang gui
Shen geng
Da zhao

Shi chun da bu tang is made with:
Ren shen
Bai zhu
Fu ling
Zhi gan cao
Shu di huang
Bai shao
Dan gui
Chuan xiong

Huang chee
Ro gui

Generally speaking, in order to prevent and treat the disease, it is necessary to remove and avoid secondary infection or to remove tumors or cancer. In addition, the patient needs proper rest, to avoid catching cold and to take in higher nutrition, such as vitamins and high protein foods.

If it is a chronic disease we can choose massage, water treatment, heat therapy, acupuncture. If it is rheumatoid multiple sclerosis then you have to see your Oriental physician or acupuncturist more frequently, because he can balance and make your body strong. Hopefully the problem will be dealt with and allow you to recover sooner.

Chapter 16

Chinese Folk Remedies for Treating Arthritis

For any of the five types of arthritis you may also use these popular Chinese Folk Remedies for treatment.

Lie down and rest, properly increase nutrition, avoid sunshine. Take it easy and don't become exhausted. Don't catch cold, and avoid other infections. Eat a lot of nourishing foods high in protein, for example, meat and fish. Increase vitamin C and E, and try to keep mentally pleasant. Meditation is very helpful.

Soak in a hot bath. Add a cup or so of Epsom salt and some 75% rubbing alcohol. Soak for 20 to 25 minutes. (If you can't stand the smell of the rubbing alcohol, use the Epsom salt only.)

Take 1 kg of salt (mountain salt, eating salt, sea salt, rock salt, any salt), and 120g of Xiao Hui Xiang (Foeniculum fructus, or **fennel**), and stir-fry. Place in a cloth bag and apply it to the painful area.

Place a wet towel in a microwave oven, and heat it up. Then put the towel in a plastic bag and apply to the painful area. You can also use the towel without the plastic bag to directly cover the painful area.

Blow directly on the painful area with a hair dryer. You can also combine with methods 2 and 3 above.

Boil 80g of willow tree branches in water, and drink the tea.

Put 30g of *Ji Gu Cao (Abria Herba)* in water. Boil. Drink the tea every day.

Take some *Huang Qi Tang (Astragalus Radix)*, sweet rice, black bean, *Long Yan Rou (Logana Arillus)*, add water, boil and drink. (People with diabetes don't use the *Long Yan Rou*).

Use self-massage or acupressure, and pound around the meridian channel with your hands. Grasp the area suddenly and release—do whatever you can to promote the energy flowing through the area.

Take a bath in Chinese herbal tea, such as:
   Dang Gui [Angelica sinensis radix]
   Chuan Xiong [Ligusticum rhizoma]
   Chang Huo, Du Huo [Angelica pubescens radix]
   Gui Zhi [Cinnamomum ramlus]
   Qin Jiao [Gentiana radix]
   Chuan Wu [Aconitum carmichaeli radix]
   Ji Gu Cao [Abri herba]
   Mu Gua [Chaenomeles fructus]
   Lu Lu Tong [Liquidambar fructus]

Hong Hua [Aarthamus flos] and
Ru Xiang [Boswellia Resin].

Drink *Shaolin* monk five fragrant wine. Soak in alcohol
for 90 days and drink:
   Ding Xiang [Eugenia caryophyllata]
   Mu Xiang [Saussurea radix]
   Tan Xiang, Xiao Hui Xiang [Foeniculum fructus]
   Dang Gui [Angelica sinensis radix]
   Chuan Xiong [Ligusticum rhizoma]
   Niu Xiss [Cyathula radix]
   Su Mu [Sappan lignum]
   Hong Hua [Aarthamus flos].

Soak the following herbs in natural vinegar:
   Ru Xiang [Boswellia resin]
   Mo Yao [Myrrh resina]
   San Qi [Pseudoginseng radix]
   Hong Hua [Aarthamus flos]
   Bo He [Mentha folium]
   Mu Xiang [Saussurea radix]
   Xue Jie [Calamus draco]

Use a cloth to soak it up, and apply to the painful area,
or rub into the skin with thumbs, hands, or even use
ginger-root to rub it on the skin.

Chapter 17

Conclusion

I hope that this book has helped you to understand more about arthritis. As I said earlier, I believe that every person has arthritis in some form, even though they may not realize it. It is very important to learn how to deal with it, since it is inevitable. However, even though it may be unavoidable, there is a lot you can do to prevent the disease from becoming a negative factor in your life.

If you already have arthritis, you can see by the material here that you do not have to continue to suffer with it. You can escape the pain. You can build up your body so that it is better able to deal with the disease.

Eastern treatment is extremely effective with all types of arthritis. You don't have to automatically succumb to the typical western methods of treatment, which in most cases are drug-related. Drugs may relieve your symptoms for awhile, but in the long run end up damaging organs and systems.

Any kind of pharmaceutical intervention leaves something undesirable behind in the body tissues. I prefer to use eastern methods, which are more natural, and do not introduce synthetic toxic materials. We must consider a person's entire body and bring it into harmony. When all the systems and organs are functioning as they should, arthritis will not be a problem.

Glossary

Acupuncture—A Chinese medical practice to treat illness or provide local anesthesia by the insertion of needles at specified sites of the body.

Amphiarthrodial Joints—Slightly moveable joints.

Articular Bones—the bones in a joint.

Articular Capsules—the structures enclosing the joints, the inside of which are lined by synovial tissue or synovial membrane.

Auscultation—To make a diagnosis by listening to the patient's body sounds.

***Bi* Syndrome**—Painful syndrome, causing both pain and weakness, relating to deficiency and/or excess.

Blood Deficiency—Clinical manifestations include pale or sallow complexion, pale lips, dizziness, poor memory, blurring of vision, palpitations, insomnia, numbness of hands and feet, a pale tongue and thready pulse.

Blood Stagnation—Manifests in symptoms such as fixed, boring or stabbing pain, mass tumors which do not move, hemorrhage with dark blood and clots, purple lips and nails, purple blotches or bruises on skin, purple tongue and wiry, choppy or knotted pulse.

Borborygmus—Intestinal rumbling caused by the movement of gas.

Cartilage—An elastic tissue on the ends of bones in a joint, which allows free movement without friction.

Chi—Energy. Also known as *qi*.

Chronic—A condition which occurs or recurs over a long period of time.

Cold—Caused by Cold Pathogenic Factor or diminished vital function, marked by intolerance of cold, fondness for warmth, loose bowels, pale tongue with coating, slow pulse, etc.

Cold in the Middle Burner—Usually refers to cold in the spleen and stomach. Marked by cold and pain over the stomach, anorexia, abdominal fullness, belching, vomiting thin fluid, diarrhea, lassitude and cold limbs.

Corticosteroid—A pharmaceutical drug used to prevent or reduce inflammation.

Dampness—Caused externally by Damp Pathogenic Factor or internally by a dysfunction of the spleen and kidney in promoting water circulation and distribution. Symptoms include heaviness in the limbs, headache as if the head were tightly bound, fullness in the chest, joint pains and swelling, diarrhea, abdominal fullness, sallow face, edema of the lower limbs, turbid discharges, etc.

Damp Heat—A combination of Dampness and Heat, which produces varying symptoms depending on the part of the body affected. Symptoms include: loss of appetite, nausea, vomiting, bitter taste and stickiness in the mouth, heaviness of the body and limbs, fullness of the chest, lassitude, jaundice, loose stools or diarrhea with blood or mucus, offensive odor of stools, burning in the anus, scanty yellow urine, abdominal pain and distention, eczema, swelling and burning pain in the testes, yellow foul-smelling leukorrhea, frequent and urgent urination, burning pain in the urethra, dribbling urination, turbid, deep yellow urine. Pulse is rapid and slippery, tongue is red with a sticky yellow coating.

Deficiency—Deficiency of vital energy and lowered body resistance. Some deficiency symptoms include emaciation, listlessness, lassitude, shortness of breath, pallor, insomnia, poor memory, spontaneous and night sweating, nocturnal enuresis, pain alleviated by pressure. Tongue is dry with little or no coating; pulse is weak and thready.

Deficiency Heat or Fire—Caused by a deficiency of *yin*, symptoms include afternoon or low grade fever, flushed cheeks, dry mouth, insomnia with mental restlessness, anxiety, feverish sensations in the palms and soles, night sweats, constipation, concentrated urine, etc. Tongue is red with little coating, pulse is rapid, thready, and empty.

Diarthrodial Joints—Freely moveable joints.

Dryness—One of the Six Pathogenic Factors which prevails in autumn or in dry climates, causing consumption of body fluids with constipation, reduced urination, etc. Also an internal condition caused by impairment of *yin*.

Essence (also known as *Jing*)—refers to the combination of the energy that makes up a person's inherited constitution and the energy derived from food. It resides mostly in the kidneys and is the basis of growth, reproduction, and development. It is also the source of kidney *qi* and of constitutional strength. Deficiency of Essence results in a variety of symptoms such as stunted growth, poor bone development or bone deterioration, infertility, habitual miscarriage, loose teeth, hair falling out or prematurely gray, poor sexual function, impotence, weakness of knees, ringing in the ears, poor memory, poor concentration, dizziness, lowered body resistance, and chronic allergies.

Etiology—The study of the causes of disease.

Exogenous—originating from outside; derived externally.

Exterior (See also Interior)—Refers to the depth of disease. Exterior syndromes are caused by invasion of the Six Pathogenic Factors, which first attack the superficial portions of the body. In general, these syndromes are of sudden onset and short duration. Chief symptoms include intolerance to cold or wind, fever, headache, nasal obstruction and superficial pulse.

Fire—A severe form of heat, manifestations include high fever, restlessness, insomnia, mania, delirium, thirst, sweating, mouth and tongue ulcers, swollen and painful gums, headache, congestion of the eyes.

Food Stagnation—Symptom pattern includes stomach pain and distention, loss of appetite, foul belching, acid regurgitation, vomiting. Tongue has a thick, sticky coating.

Gout—a form of osteoarthritis, most often affecting the great toe. It is a painful inflammation due to an excess of uric acid in the blood.

Heart Blood Deficiency—Symptom pattern includes giddiness, pallor, palpitation, insomnia, forgetfulness, fine and weak pulse.

Heart Qi Deficiency—Symptom pattern includes palpitation, shortness of breath on exertion, spontaneous sweating, fine, weak or irregular pulse.

Heart Yin Deficiency—Symptom pattern includes mental irritability, palpitation, insomnia, low fever, night sweat, flushed cheeks, thirst, fine, rapid pulse.

Heat—Caused by Pathogenic Heat or by excessive vital function. Marked by feverishness, flushed face, thirst, craving for cold drinks, constipation, red tongue with yellow coating, rapid pulse.

Heat in the Blood—marked by restlessness or mania, feeling of heat, skin diseases with red eruptions, mouth ulcers, itching, excessive menstrual bleeding hemorrhage, dry mouth, red tongue, rapid pulse.

Heat Toxin—Refers to toxic heat generated by bacterial or viral infection.

Inflammation—Redness, swelling or fever, often accompanied by pain.

Interior (See also Exterior)—Refers to the depth of the disease. Interior syndromes are mostly severe or chronic and deep. In interior diseases the pathogenic factors are on the interior of the body and attack the organs.

Jing (see Essence)

Kidney Yang Deficiency—Symptom pattern includes pallor, cold limbs, soreness and weakness of the lumbar region and knee joints, nocturnal urination, impotence, infertility, dizziness, ringing in the ears, a pale tongue with white coating, a deep, weak pulse.

Kidney Yin Deficiency—Symptom pattern includes: low back pain, weak knees, lassitude, general weakness, vertigo, ringing in the ears, thirst, flushed cheeks, mental irritability, afternoon fever, night sweats, nocturnal emission, yellow urine, constipation, red tongue with little coating, thready, rapid pulse.

Liver Blood Deficiency—Symptom pattern includes: sallow face, blurring of vision, dry eyes, spasms of muscles and tendons, dizziness, mental irritability, insomnia, absent or scanty menstruation, prolonged menstrual cycle, pale tongue or lips.

Liver Fire—Symptom pattern includes dizziness, headache, flushed face, red eyes, bitter taste in the mouth, mental irritability, and angry outbursts. In severe cases symptoms include: mania, nosebleed, blood in the urine, or coughing blood. Tongue is scarlet red on tip and sides, with yellow coating. Pulse is wiry and rapid.

Liver Heat—Marked by mental irritability, bitter taste in mouth, thirst, etc. Similar to Fire but not as severe.

Liver Qi Stagnation—Manifests in irritability, tendency to anger, dizziness, abdominal and hypochondriac pain and distention, fullness in chest, excessive sighing, breast distention, belching, loss of appetite, nausea, sensation of a foreign body in throat, menstrual disorders.

Liver/Spleen Disharmony—Symptom pattern includes abdominal pain and distention, diarrhea or loose stools, belching, vomiting, acid regurgitation.

Liver Wind—Usually resulting from Liver Fire or Deficient Blood. Symptoms include dizziness and vertigo, convulsions, tremors, spasms and numbness.

Liver Yang Rising—Manifests in headache with distending sensation in the head, dizziness and vertigo, ringing in the ears, flushed face, red eyes, irritability, insomnia with dream-disturbed sleep, palpitations, poor memory, red tongue and a tight and rapid pulse.

Liver Yin Deficiency—Symptom pattern includes dizziness, headache, ringing in the ears, blurred vision, dry eyes, insomnia, night sweats, feverishness in palms and soles, thirst, dry throat. Pulse is thready and taut. Tongue is reddened with little coating.

Low Burner—Refers to the "lower" organs of kidneys, bladder and large intestine.

Lung Heat—Marked by cough with thick or yellow phlegm, pain in the chest, and shortness of breath.

Lung *Yin* Deficiency—Manifests in symptoms such as dry or blood tinged cough, or cough with a small amount of sticky sputum, dryness of the mouth and throat, afternoon fever, flushed cheeks, night sweats, feverishness in palms and soles. Tongue is red with little coating. Pulse is thready and rapid.

Meridians—The ascending and descending pathways or channels which are connected to all internal structures, systems, and organs.

Middle Burner—Refers usually to the "middle" organs of spleen and stomach.

Middle Qi Deficiency—Refers to deficiency of *qi* of the spleen and stomach, resulting in hypo-function of those organs, digestive disorders, weakness, etc. (See Spleen and Stomach *Qi* Deficiency).

Moxibustion—Used in conjunction with acupuncture, it is a procedure where mugwort, an herb, is burned on or near the acupuncture points to stimulate them.

Neuro-area Disease—Disease relating to the central nervous system or nerves.

Normal *Qi*—Body energy made up of *Qi* inherited from parents, *Qi* from food, and *Qi* from air. Responsible for the movement, functioning and warmth of the body and for protection from disease.

NSAIDS—Nonsteroidal anti-inflammatory drugs often used in the treatment of arthritis.

Olfaction—A method of diagnosis using smell.

Osteoblast—Bone forming cell.

Osteoclast—Bone absorbing cell.

Osteophyte—Abnormal growth of cartilage and bone, or bone spur.

Painful Obstruction—Obstruction of vital energy and blood flow, usually bringing on pains, specifically arthritis, due to Wind, Cold and Dampness blocking the channels of the limbs.

Palpation—a method of diagnosis in which any pathological condition is detected by palpating, feeling and pressing certain areas of the body to learn of local abnormal changes. This method is divided into two categories: pulse taking, and touching different parts of the body.

Pathogen—Any disease-producing agent.

Pathology—The science or study of the origin, nature, and course of diseases, or the conditions and processes of a disease.

Pathogenic Factors—The causes of disease. Pathogenic Factors include Wind, Cold, Dampness, Heat, Dryness, and Fire. These can be of exterior origin (related to extreme or sudden climatic changes such as invasion by Wind-Cold) or they can be internally generated such as Liver-Wind.

Periosteum—The layer of fibrous connective tissue covering the outer shell of bone.

Philosophy—A system of principles for guidance in practical affairs.

Phlegm—Results from an accumulation of bodily fluids due to a dysfunction of the lung, spleen and kidney and impairment of water metabolism. Clinical manifestations are many and vary depending on the area of the body affected. Symptoms can include cough with profuse sputum, asthmatic breathing, fullness in the chest, palpitations, coma, manic-depressive disorders, lymph node swelling, nodules under the skin, dizziness, blurred vision, sensation of a foreign body in the throat, edema, general body aching and heaviness, nausea, vomiting of sticky fluid, borborygmus, stomach and abdominal discomfort.

Phlegm Heat—Often seen in Lung or Stomach Patterns, clinical manifestations include yellow-sticky phlegm, barking cough with profuse yellow or green sputum, fullness in the chest, asthma, dry mouth and lips, restlessness. Tongue is red with a sticky, yellow coating. Pulse is rapid and slippery.

Physiology—The organic processes or functions in an organism or its parts.

Protective (See Wei Qi)

Resorption—The dissolution or assimilation of a substance, such as bone tissue.

Qi—Energy, also known as chi.

Qi Deficiency—Symptoms include: general weakness, lethargy, shortness of breath, weak voice, spontaneous sweating, loss of appetite, abdominal distention, loose stools, frequent urination, palpitations and an empty pulse.

Scleroderma—A form of arthritis in which connective tissues become hardened and rigid.

Spleen Dampness—Symptoms include lack of appetite, sticky taste in the mouth or loss of sense of taste, nausea, fullness in the chest and abdomen, feeling of heaviness, loose stools, headache as if head were bound. Tongue has sticky coating. Pulse is slippery.

Spleen Qi Deficiency—Clinical manifestations include sallow complexion, emaciation, tiredness, dislike of speaking, reduced appetite, abdominal distention, loose stools, prolapse. Tongue is pale with a thin white coating. Pulse is empty, weak, or thready.

Spleen *Yang* Deficiency—Symptom pattern includes pallor, cold limbs, poor appetite, abdominal distension which is worse after eating, dull abdominal pain which improves with warmth and pressure, loose stools. Tongue is pale with a white coating. Pulse is deep and slow.

Stomach Phlegm—Symptoms include nausea, vomiting of sticky fluid, stomach and abdominal fullness and discomfort, borborygmus. Tongue coating is sticky and pulse is slippery.

Stomach *Qi* Deficiency—Clinical manifestations include an uncomfortable feeling in the stomach, no appetite, lack of taste sensation, loose stools, tiredness, especially in the morning, weak limbs. Tongue is pale. Pulse is weak and empty, especially in the middle position of the right hand.

Synovial Fluid—Lubricating fluid found inside joints which aids in smooth movement.

Synovial Membrane—The lining of moveable joints which secretes synovial fluid.

Summer Heat—One of the Six Pathogenic Factors. Pathogenic Summer Heat is caused by prolonged exposure to blazing sun on hot days or too much time in a hot room with poor ventilation. Summer Heat consumes *Qi* and *Yin* and may disturb the mind. Symptoms include excessive sweating, thirst, shortness of breath, lassitude, concentrated urine and in extreme cases, fever, restlessness, red, dry skin, and delirium or coma. May combine with Damp to produce dizziness, heaviness in the head, stifling sensation in the chest, nausea, poor appetite, diarrhea, and general sluggishness.

Synarthrodial Joints—Immobile joints.

Tinnitus—A sensation of ringing in the ears.

Tophi—Small stones or crystals, sometimes present in a joint affected with gout, or on the outer surface of the ear.

Unstable or Disturbed *Shen*—*Shen* is translated as "Spirit." It refers to the mind, consciousness, the force of the personality, and the connection to the spiritual aspects of humanness. When *Shen* is disturbed or unstable, symptoms arise such as insomnia, unclear or muddled thinking, poor memory, restlessness, hysteria, incoherent speech, delirium, mania.

Wei *Qi*—Refers to defensive energy, which protects the body from invasion by external pathogenic factors.

Wei Syndrome—a syndrome relating to excess, where muscles and/or tendons have atrophied, causing tendons and meridians to become flaccid and soft. Generally speaking in *wei* syndrome, there is no pain, only weakness.

Wen—auscultation and olfaction (listening and smelling) together make up one entity in diagnosis known as *wen*.

Wind—One of the six Pathogenic Factors. External Wind is usually combined with one of the other pathogenic factors (Cold, Heat, Dampness, and Dryness) which depend on wind to invade the body. Symptoms of External Wind include headache, stiff neck, nasal obstruction, sneezing, itching or skin rash, joint pains, and superficial pulse. Internal or Endogenous Wind causes symptoms such as headaches, stiff neck, irritability, dizziness, fainting, high fever, delirium, coma, convulsions, tremor, tics, blurred vision, numbness, facial paralysis, and wandering pains.

Wind-Cold—Symptoms include aversion to cold, shivering, sneezing, cough, runny nose with watery or white discharge, slight fever or no fever, neck pain and stiffness, no sweating. Pulse is tight and superficial. Tongue looks normal (normal color, thin white coating).

Wind-Heat—Symptoms are similar to those above except with symptoms of heat such as fever, yellow mucus, sore throat, swollen tonsils, thirst, sweating. Pulse is floating and rapid. Tongue is red on the tip or sides, with a thin, white or yellowish coating.

Wind-Damp—Symptoms include itchy skin, rashes, hives, fever, aversion to cold, sweating, neck pain and stiffness, body aches and heaviness, swollen joints. Pulse is superficial and slippery.

Yang Qi—Warming, energy, positive *qi*.

Yin and Yang—Two principles, one negative, dark, and feminine (*yin*) and one positive, bright, and masculine (*yang*) whose interaction influences the destinies of creatures and things.

Yuan Qi—your body's foundation, made up of your inherited constitution plus *gu qi* (fuel) and atmosphere *qi* (air) to your kidney essence.

Zang / Fu Organs—The body has six *zang* and six *fu* organs: Zang organs mainly work at night; *fu* organs work during the day. Zang Organs are: Liver, Heart, Spleen, Lung, Kidney. Fu Organs are: Large intestine, Stomach, Small intestine, Urinary bladder, Triple warmer, Gall bladder

Zang Qi Insufficient—Immune system is weak.

The Four Great Medical Books in TCM

1. Huang Di Nei Jing. The Yellow Emperor's Internal Classic, or **Canon of Medicine**. Same book, but different name, two portions: (a) Su Wen/"Plain Questions," (b) Ling Shu/"Miraculous Pivot." Compiled: Western Han (206BC-8AD). Contents: a. Prevention of diseases, b. Treatment, c. Anatomy, d. Circulation.

2. Nan Jing. *Difficult Classic*, compiled or appeared at 1st-2nd Century BC. Contents are a. Fundamental medical theories & expounds the main points of Nei Jing; b. Points of Acupuncture & Moxibustion; c. Method of Pulsing.

3. Shang Han Za Bing Lun. The *Treatise on Febrile & Miscellaneous Diseases*, author Dr. Zhang Zhong-Jing, rearranged by Dr. Wang Shu who divided it into: *The Bureau for Censoring & Publishing Medical Books:* a. Shang Han Lun; b. Jin Kui Yao Lue Fang Lun/Jin Kui Yao Lue. Compiled at the beginning of the 3rd Century AD. Contents are diagnosis and treatment of fevers and other miscellaneous diseases.

4. <u>Shen Nong Ben Cao Jing</u>. *Shen Nong's Herbal,* Author Unknown, attributed to ancient emperor Shen Nong. Arranged by Dr. Tao Hung-Ching (540 AD). Compiled: Believed to be in the 1st Century. Contents are 365 herbs listed, which are divided into three classes, such as superior, common and inferior.

References

Kaptchuk, Ted J. The Web That Has No Weaver. Chicago: Congdon, 1983.

Lu, Gwei-Djen, and Joseph Needham. Medicine in Traditional China. Recent Advances in Traditional Medicine in East Asia. Eds. Toshitsugu Oda, Joseph Needham, Yasuo Otsuka, and Liu Guo-bin. Tokyo: Excerpta Medica, 1985.

Pálos, Stephan. The Chinese Art of Healing. Trans. William Gutman. New York: Herder, 1971.

Teresawa, Katsutoshi. The Role of Traditional Chinese Medicine in Contemporary Health Care in Japan.

Tiang, Jingfu. Traditional Chinese Medicine. Wu, Hsien-Chung et al. Creating a New Chinese Medicine and Pharmacology. Beijing: Foreign Language Press, 1977.

Wu, Hsien-Chung et al. Creating a New Chinese Medicine and Pharmacology. Beijing: Foreign Language Press, 1977.

Zhong-Jing, Zhang, Shang Han Za Bing Lun. Treatise on Febrile & Miscellaneous Diseases, rearranged by Dr. Wang Shu. Compiled at Beginning of 3rd Century AD. Contents: Diagnosis and treatment of fevers and other miscellaneous diseases.

Printed in the United Kingdom
by Lightning Source UK Ltd.
104219UKS00001B/110